*Praise for Inna Segal's*

# THE SECRET LANGUAGE

## OF YOUR BODY

This book has received international support from a wide range
of prominent doctors, nurses, psychologists, bestselling authors,
and natural health practitioners.

"*The Secret Language of Your Body* truly is the essential guide to restoring your body to its healthiest state and assist you to heal your life. Inna Segal offers invaluable insights into the underlying causes of illness and disease and provides practical advice, which will undoubtedly empower many to self-heal. So, read on and learn from the wisdom of this book, which can guide you to the life you were truly meant to live."
—**Bernie S. Siegel, MD**, *New York Times* bestselling author of *Love, Medicine & Miracles*

"*The Secret Language of Your Body* is thrilling and right on target! My fondest hope is that people all over the planet will take this message of healing into their hearts and bodies, and become vibrantly well!"
—**Christiane Northrup, MD**, *New York Times* bestselling author of
*Women's Bodies, Women's Wisdom*

"*The Secret Language of Your Body* teaches you how to listen to the messages your body gives, and leads you step-by-step to create great health through simple but effective healing methods and principles. Inna Segal explains and demonstrates how your thoughts, energy, and emotions affect your health, so your body's wisdom won't be a secret anymore but a powerful guide to transform every area of your life."
—**Jack Canfield**, coauthor of the *Chicken Soup for the Soul*® series
and author of *The Success Principles*™

"An easy-to-use practical guide for establishing a relationship with your own body and its healing potential, this book offers you user-friendly tools to participate in your own healing. *The Secret Language of Your Body* is an inspiring guide for learning to communicate effectively with our own bodies."

—**Brandon Bays**, bestselling author of *The Journey*

"You don't have to be ill to benefit from this remarkable book. Ms. Segal provides simple but powerful exercises that help you connect with your body and inner wisdom to promote physical, mental, and emotional healing at the deepest level, allowing you to live a happy, healthy, and more abundant life."

—**Hyla Cass, MD**, author of *Natural Highs* and former assistant clinical professor of Psychiatry at UCLA School of Medicine

"I was a skeptic at first look. But I tried it and discovered this to be a magical book. Quite simply, it works and it can heal you."

—**Roger Cole, MD**, cancer and palliative care specialist, and bestselling author of *Mission of Love*

"Even if you don't know what's wrong with you yet, this book helps you start on the road to healing and—with the guidance of Inna—eventually even a cure!"

—**Jerry M. Rosenbaum, MD**, coauthor of *What's Wrong with Me?*

"*Livid, pissed off, torn up inside, heartache, bone weary, jaundiced, gut wrenching, blood boiling, pain in the neck, stab in the back, take my breath away, rash decision, sick to death*—our language is alive with ancient wisdom about the origin of many illnesses. *The Secret Language of Your Body* allows you to recognize and set yourself free from the toxic effects of unconscious beliefs and emotions, and start on a path of self-healing."

—**Robin Youngson, MD**, founder of the Centre for Compassion in Healthcare

"I have used many of the processes and the improvements in my quality of life are truly remarkable."

—**Mary-Anne Gallagher**, registered psychologist

"An amazing book from a renowned healer. Think of it as the Introduction Manual for ultra health of the mind, body, and spirit."

—**Siimon Reynolds**, chairman/creative director of Love Communications and author of *Become Happy in Eight Minutes*

"Inna shows us how to read and communicate with our body. She has beautifully managed to tap into what is possibly the next frontier for psychologists: the wisdom that our amazing bodies have for us. This book is full of useful insights into ourselves and, more importantly, into ways for living holistically."

—**Rob Hilliar**, registered psychologist

"Inna's detailed book will help you gain a more profound understanding of the intimacies of the mind–body connection. Her brilliant insights and compelling case histories challenge all of us to transcend our preconceptions and personal limitations."

—**Dr. Con Rallis**, chiropractor

"A great set of insights into how to stay healthy and well!"

—**Thom Hartmann**, bestselling author of *Cracking the Code* and host of *The Thom Hartmann Program* on KPOJ Radio

"Our health is a key element of living a successful life. *The Secret Language of Your Body* explores and develops your awareness of the important mind, body, and spirit connection that is vital to living a healthy life."

—**Jim Stovall**, bestselling author of *The Ultimate Gift*

"Inna Segal's advice and techniques are spot-on when it comes to effectiveness. As a practitioner with many years experience in healing therapies, I can vouch for the accuracy and practicality of Inna's recommendations. I recommend you buy this book. It is set to become a classic in the field of mind–body medicine."

—**Dr. Ralph Ballard**, MBBS, Dip Hom, Dip Clinical Hypnosis

"With her book *The Secret Language of Your Body*, Inna Segal has made a significant contribution to the growing body of knowledge in the field of mind–body–spirit. Her work encompasses the underlying mental and emotional causes of malfunction in all parts of the body, with additional insights into emotions and the use of color in healing. Importantly, her book focuses on what people can do for themselves rather than what healthcare professionals can do for them."

—**Peter Johnston**, holistic general practitioner

"Discover your inner intelligence and transform your life! This is the potential of Inna Segal's book. *The Secret Language of Your Body* is a well-written, practical, and insightful do-it-yourself guide for healing any health problem using one's own intuition. It may be just the guide you need on your journey to wellness."

—**Tim Bajraszewski, MD**, general practitioner

"Inna has intuitively given a comprehensive and practical explanation of life's problems and their treatment. *The Secret Language of Your Body* is a great book for those seeking love, inner peace, and whole-body integration."

—**Shaun Resnik, ND**, naturopath and homeopath

"Inna's book on the underlying and energetic causes of illness is one of the most comprehensive texts of its kind. Inna writes with a style that makes this important information easily accessible to anyone who wants to learn about the emotional contribution to disease. Especially powerful are the meditations provided, making this book not only a great source of insight but essentially practical as well."

—**Darren Walsh, BHS (Acu)**, doctor of Chinese medicine

"Inna is an amazingly gifted healer. I have partaken in two workshops, which have had a profound effect on my life. Inna opened doors for me that created the opportunity to grow, learn, and understand how to heal myself and others. *The Secret Language of Your Body* is an excellent, understandable, easy guide to changing your life for the better."

—**Jo Hill, RN**

# The
# Secret
# Language
## of your
# Body

# THE
# SECRET
# LANGUAGE
## OF YOUR
# BODY

## THE ESSENTIAL GUIDE TO
## HEALTH AND WELLNESS

# INNA SEGAL
### FOREWORD BY BERNIE S. SIEGEL, MD

**ATRIA** PAPERBACK
New York London Toronto Sydney New Delhi

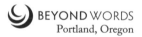
BEYOND WORDS
Portland, Oregon

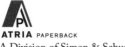

**ATRIA** PAPERBACK
A Division of Simon & Schuster, Inc.
1230 Avenue of the Americas
New York, NY 10020

BEYOND WORDS
1750 S.W. Skyline Blvd., Suite 20
Portland, OR 97221-2543
503-531-8700 / 503-531-8773 fax
www.beyondword.com

Managing editor: Lindsay S. Brown
Editor: Jenefer Angell-Mros
Copyeditor: Henry Covey
Proofreader: Jennifer Weaver-Neist
Design: Devon Smith
Composition: William H. Brunson Typography Services

First Atria Paperback/Beyond Words trade paperback edition August 2010

**ATRIA** PAPERBACK and colophon are trademarks of Simon & Schuster, Inc.
Beyond Words Publishing is a division of Simon & Schuster, Inc.

For more information about special discounts for bulk purchases,
please contact Simon & Schuster Special Sales at 1-866-506-1949
or business@simonandschuster.com.

The Simon & Schuster Speakers Bureau can bring authors to your live event.
For more information or to book an event, contact the Simon & Schuster Speakers
Bureau at 1-866-248-3049 or visit our website at www.simonspeakers.com.

Manufactured in the United States of America

30

*Library of Congress Cataloging-in-Publication Data*

Segal, Inna.
    The secret language of your body : the essential guide to health and wellness / Inna Segal ; foreword by
 Bernie S. Siegel. — 1st Atria Pbk./Beyond Words trade pbk. ed.
        p.    cm.
    Includes index.
    1. Mental health.    2. Mental healing.    3. Self-care, Health.    I. Title.
    RA790.S4525    2010
    616.89—dc22
                                                                            2010009561

ISBN 978-1-58270-260-5
ISBN 971-1-4391-7671-9 (ebook)

The corporate mission of Beyond Words Publishing, Inc.: *Inspire to Integrity*

This book rests in the hands of Divinity
and is dedicated to the Infinite Love
within us all.

The Secret Language of Your Body is more than a book,
it is part of a new healthcare movement, encouraging and
teaching people to tune into their own bodies and participate
in their self-healing.

This is an interactive experience
containing powerful processes and healing frequencies
to lead people to greater health and wellness.

# CONTENTS

# ACKNOWLEDGMENTS

Firstly, I would like to thank my husband, Ty. You have rocked my whole world and changed my life more than I could ever imagine was possible. You constantly inspire and challenge me to refine and walk the path of truth. Every day with you is magical! Let's keep supporting each other to help move humanity forward.

I thank my children, Raphael and Angelina, for their love. You allow my heart to grow and give me deep joy and appreciation for the important things in life.

I am grateful to my parents, Lena and Kolia, who always encourage me in my healing, writing, and teaching. I am very proud of my mum, who has attended all my courses and read all my articles. It touches my heart to see you change through the Divine healing and wisdom you have discovered within yourself. You are amazing.

I would also like to thank everyone in my family, especially my brother, Marat, who is a very loving and helpful brother. You are always there when I need you, and I deeply appreciate having you in my life. I love you.

To my beautiful cousin, Jenny, thank you for your enthusiasm, encouragement, and willingness to listen. I love sharing my journey with you; watching you change, grow, and become the Divine, empowered, magnificent person I know you to be. I love you, appreciate you, and am inspired by you.

To my grandparents, Emma and Misha, thank you for showing me what it means to be courageous and to fight for life. I am so blessed to have you in my life.

# ACKNOWLEDGMENTS

I would like to thank Dr. Levent Efe, a medical illustrator, for his artistic skill and understanding of the human body. It was a pleasure working with you.

I also thank my clients and workshop participants. Being open enough to try the healing processes I teach gives me the opportunity to have the best job in the world—not the easiest, but definitely the most fulfilling. I can think of nothing better than to watch people transform in front of my eyes.

To my close friends, Marina and Sarah, thank you for bringing fun, laughter, and joy into my life. I am so happy to know that you are there for me.

To my amazing friend, Piotr, thank you for your unconditional love, patience, and encouragement. My life will never be the same again. Thank you for designing beautiful clothes for me.

I would like to thank my ex husband Paul Segal for all the support you gave me while I was writing this book, working with clients, and traveling the world.

To Adam Jones, an incredible fashion designer and close friend, you are one of the funniest and most generous people I know. Thank you to Faye Wenke for your belief in my work and for recommending this book to Beyond Words Publishing.

A special thank you to Cynthia Black of Beyond Words Publishing for your encouragement and enthusiasm and to Judith Curr at Atria Books for all your support and belief in me. Thank you to the rest of the team at Beyond Words: Richard Cohn, Tim Schroeder, Jenefer Angell-Mros, Lindsay S. Brown, Devon Smith, Georgie Lewis, Jessica Sturges, and Whitney Quon. Working with the Beyond Words team has been an absolute dream come true. I have been touched, inspired, and expanded by your love, care, and dedication. Thank you from the depth of my heart.

After many years of exploring and searching, I have been deeply inspired by the brilliance of Rudolf Steiner. I deeply encourage anyone who is open minded and open hearted to explore the work of this truly outstanding man and the incredible gifts he brought to humanity.

# FOREWORD

*The Secret Language of Your Body* is what the subtitle says it is: The Essential Guide. You are then likely to ask: But why do I need a guide, and what am I being guided to? My response would be that this book can guide you to the life you were truly meant to live, which the majority of us are not living. Each Monday morning, we have more suicides, strokes, illnesses, and heart attacks. I think our bodies are trying very hard to tell us something about how our lives, jobs, relationships, and attitudes affect our bodies and our health.

If we do not pay attention to our feelings and the messages from our bodies, then our bodies will assume we do not enjoy life and get us out of here as quickly as possible. I think that is the message of this book—to stop living your untrue self's life, which others have imposed upon you, and to eliminate not yourself but what is killing you. Thus, by paying attention to the messages from within your body, you're saving your life.

*The Secret Language of Your Body* is practical and oriented to your life and time. So, read on and be guided to a new life by words you can understand and actions you can perform; be born again and restore your body to its healthiest state, letting *it* guide *you* to heal your life.

A healed life carries many benefits, one of which can be a cured disease. Just as bacteria, viruses, and plants alter their genetic makeup to resist antibiotics, vaccines, and weather changes, we are capable of inner healing too. It is a lot harder for us because our lives are a lot more complicated, but if we listen to the messages from our intelligent cells and create an internal environment which nurtures life, then self-induced healing can become a more frequent occurrence.

But first, you must be willing to pay attention to your body and feelings and not live solely in your head and thoughts. Distractions and drugs are not the proper response to your feelings. As a lawyer once said in a time of crisis (and lawyering can be a serious illness), "I came to a conclusion that was imminently reasonable, totally logical, and completely wrong because, while learning to think, I almost forgot how to feel."

The reason most people have a hard time paying attention to their feelings is because their feelings are painful. The majority of people grow up with mottos to die by rather than live by. They need to abandon their painful pasts and get over the destructive messages received from various authority figures, such as parents, teachers, clergy, doctors, and others.

The effect of words upon children up to the age of six is hypnotic and very difficult to overcome as they grow older and begin to feel the destructive toll upon their bodies and health. Often, the search for better feelings leads to violent behavior and a variety of addictions as the result of their damaged nervous systems. The language of your body doesn't have to remain a secret. We do not want you to awaken to life and become strong at the broken places from the result of a major disaster. We would like you to learn from your body how to survive and be strong enough to stand up to the forces of nature while still supple enough to bend when circumstances require it. By bringing meaning to your symptoms, you can be guided to heal.

Pain is necessary for us to protect and define ourselves. If we never experienced pain, it would be a disaster for our lives and bodies. But when we give the pain or affliction meaning, we do not have to suffer. Pain and suffering are two distinct entities.

Consciousness is nonlocal, and we need to tune into the messages we are receiving. Since organ recipients can tell you about the lives of their donors, we must realize our life is stored within us and our cells.

Several years ago, I developed vertigo while training for a marathon and doing all the other things I normally do. I asked myself how I would describe this feeling to others, and the words I heard were, "The world is spinning around." I knew my body was telling me to slow down and rest; it was making it hard for me to get out of bed in the morning. When I looked up "vertigo" in this book's list of ailments, I read the same thing my body had been telling me. I am having right ankle problems at the present time, too, and when I looked it up in part I, there was the answer: "having too many responsibilities." We can talk to our bodies and learn from them, and also learn from the wisdom of this book to make it even easier and quicker to heal.

If you are willing to rehearse and practice, you can become the person you want to be. We can coach and guide you, but you have to show up for practice. We know that your blood chemistry is changed by the role you play. Even actors experience changes in their immune functions and cortisol levels when performing in a play; a tragedy can lead to illness, while a comedy can help them resist disease. Remember, we are talking about healing your life. Healing and curing are separate entities, but a healed life resists many illnesses and is more likely to lead to a cured body.

Do not let your beliefs get in the way. Let your experience be what guides you. I have learned from my body and the work of healers that amazing things can be accomplished that were never taught to me or discussed in medical school. If you live the way Inna Segal is suggesting in this book, you become a "respant." That is, you are no longer a submissive, long-suffering patient but a "responsible participant." Let the child within come forth and experience love and humor, and feel what it does for your body. My wife, Bobbie, and I used to give presentations together: she would do stand-up comedy and I would lecture on health. What impressed me was how much healthier everyone's bodies looked after fifteen minutes of laughter. And she received more thanks when we were done than I did.

So learn from your body and your problem, and let the charcoal under pressure become a diamond that frees you from the darkness and disability. I must mention that despite what many of us are brought up to believe, this is not about guilt, shame, and blame. This is not about what you did wrong but about what you can do right by participating in your life and communicating with the wisdom within you. Yes, I have been injured and developed health problems that were not about emotional issues but from things like accidents and tick bites. However, by listening to my body, I can help myself to heal more rapidly and avoid chronic problems; I do not need a disease to get my needs met. So, stop worrying about doing it right or failing because of messages from your past, and start participating in your life and playing as well as you can.

The body is our gift. It demonstrates what our lives are about, just as a television screen shows you the content of the program being viewed. I work with patients' dreams and drawings, and I know that the body communicates in symbols too. I use them to help make diagnoses so that patients can see their inner wisdom displayed and make therapeutic choices.

The colors used in patients' drawings also carry meaning and express emotions. Art therapists and Jungian therapists are aware of this, though it is not mentioned in medical school. It is no accident that Aleksandr Solzhenitsyn describes self-induced healing in his book *Cancer Ward* as "a rainbow-colored butterfly." There you have the symbol of transformation and all the emotions associated with it in one symbol. Do not be afraid to step forward and listen to your body.

This is not about doing it right or wrong, being good or bad; it is about being open to the universal language of the spirit and unconscious as spoken through our bodies. Let your body help guide you to the right choices and treatment, and ultimately the self-healing of your life too.

Bernie S. Siegel, MD
Bestselling author of *Love, Medicine & Miracles* and *Faith, Hope & Healing*

# INTRODUCTION

Learn to heal yourself and release negative beliefs that keep you imprisoned. Let go of destructive emotions, such as resentment, fear, depression, anger, failure, jealousy, and hopelessness. Connect to the wisdom of your body; learn to use your intuition; open your heart; and experience joy, compassion, clarity, relaxation, and love. Discover your body's innate intelligence and use it to create amazing transformations.

How do I know that all this is possible? I myself have experienced an incredible healing transformation and have worked with thousands of others who have changed their lives from suppression, illness, and dissatisfaction to openness, health, and the joy of intimately and profoundly knowing themselves. When you let go of the shell that covers your true nature, you discover the radiance of your authentic Self.

You don't have to believe me. This is not about listening to others but about discovering your own answers. As I tell people during my events, I believe every person who participates receives numerous gifts; many insights; expanded awareness; and opportunities for growth, transformation, and healing. What I teach gives people the key; how you use it is entirely your choice. Only you have the power to change your life.

Your body is a feedback system. This book gives you the opportunity to understand the messages your body sends you and offers a range of practical exercises to create harmony and healing. All the exercises are simple, easy, and fast; you don't need previous experience. If you can breathe, relax, read, think, and move your body, you can heal.

I have worked with many people, using these simple exercises to successfully heal a multitude of conditions: headaches, back pain, anxiety, heart problems, weight issues, digestive disorders, and asthma, to name just a few.

In your hands, you hold the tools that will clear destructive patterns, beliefs, and emotional baggage at a cellular level in order for you to discover the incredible being you really are—full of shining potential, genius, empowerment, and Divinity. All you have to do is be willing to use the information you have at your fingertips to heal yourself and change your life.

One of my students shared with me that she had never believed that she was capable of freeing herself from the despair and depression she felt until she discovered that, underneath her issues, there was a deep, profound, transformational love. Through this healing, she changed her life and her relationship with her husband, children, and family. She learned that she is loveable, and she no longer suffers from anxiety, panic attacks, depression, or heart palpitations.

Another client realized that her addiction to smoking was a way to feel closer to her father. When she recognized this, her addiction lost all its power. She stopped smoking that day.

Throughout history, many great masters, healers, and visionaries have said, "Know thyself" because when you have awareness, you have choice, and when you have choice, you have freedom and access to well-being. "Know thyself" and "heal thyself" are great concepts. The problem is that most people don't know how to do it. My intention in writing this book is to give you the tools to look within and discover the untapped fountain of wellness and vitality that we all possess.

A highly successful businessman once shared with me that learning how to tune in to his body and follow its guidance not only healed his painful back and knees but helped him make winning business decisions. In fact, after attending some of my seminars, his income tripled because of his newly enhanced, intuitive business acumen.

Discovering your inner wisdom and tuning in to yourself is not something you do a few times a year; it is a way of life. Once you begin to feel the amazing benefits, expand your awareness, and experience the power of self-healing, you will never want to turn back.

## How It All Began

As I was growing up, if someone had told me I would discover powerful healing techniques, create a new healing modality, and share it on television, in workshops, and in books, I would have thought they were crazy. My dream was to become an actress and an author. I studied acting, appeared in plays while still at school, and then studied professional writing and editing in college. I never imagined that one day I would travel internationally, empowering people to transform their lives by renewing their health and vitality.

However, maybe it's not so surprising, as health has been a reoccurring theme in my life since childhood. I was born in Minsk, the capital of Belarus, which was affected by the Chernobyl disaster. Two years after the nuclear reactor contaminated the area, doctors informed my parents that my younger brother, Marat, who had been very ill, could die from the harsh climate we lived in and the city's lack of available treatment. We made plans to move to Australia, and during the extremely stressful immigration process, we lived in Italy for nine months. The Italians were very nice to us, and there were also a lot of Russian-speaking immigrants around. Even though my parents were worried about our future, I loved my time in Italy and learned how to be independent by selling products on the beach to help my parents earn money.

Newly settled in Australia, my family had the challenge of starting a new life from scratch: learning a foreign language, adjusting to a different culture, and finding a way to survive. This difficult period had a considerable effect on my health. I became nervous, and I found it hard to express myself at school and at home. I frequently experienced severe stomach pains, skin problems, anxiety, and occasional panic attacks. At that time, my parents and grandparents believed that only doctors knew how to heal medical issues, so I was sent to them regularly.

My health continued to decline. At the age of sixteen, I began to suffer occasional but intense backaches, and a doctor referred me to a physical therapist. Despite some small initial relief, my back deteriorated to a point where my pain had became almost unbearable.

At eighteen, I met my future husband, Paul, in an acting class. Paul introduced me to a wide range of therapies. I tried an array of holistic and medical practitioners, but nothing seemed to work. I would feel slightly better for a short time, but then the pain returned and got gradually worse each time.

By age twenty, I felt so bad that for weeks I was barely able to walk. Self-conscious, I tried to hide this from my friends and family. Only Paul and my mum knew the extent of my pain. At one point, I felt like I was living at my chiropractor's office. My confidence was pretty low.

## The Turning Point

I was in agony, and my body felt and looked disfigured. I asked Paul to drive me to the chiropractor, and I screamed the whole way. Every bump in the road felt like torture.

Finally, I made it into the chiropractor's waiting room. He took one look at me and told me that my body was stuck. I stared, bewildered, and murmured, "I already know this. What are you going to do about it?"

"Nothing," he said. "Go home."

On the drive back, I was absolutely furious, and this somehow made the pain less agonizing. I have read that when a person is depressed and feels hopeless, anger can be beneficial to move them forward. I was experiencing something like that. In my mind, I was playing out various scenarios of not being able to walk or ending up in a wheelchair. Then a thought occurred to me: my health could not stay the same. It would either get worse or it would get better. The idea of enduring the pain for the rest of my life was unbearable.

Later, at home on my bed, as I contemplated my bleak future, I had an epiphany. In an incredible shift in consciousness, I realized I had always relied on others to heal me, thinking that they could somehow save me. The more I gave away my inner power, the worse I felt. The answer was clear: I needed to heal myself. But how?

## Discovering My Ability to Heal

I suddenly had a sense that my body was endowed with an incredible ability to heal. Before self-healing, however, I had to discover the purpose of my pain. Something was obviously not working, and my body was attempting to give me a message.

Even though I was still in pain, I now felt I had a purpose. I didn't know exactly how to begin self-healing, but I was aware that a human being functions on different levels—mental, emotional, physical, spiritual, energetic, and others. I decided to explore all the aspects I could.

First, I made a decision to become well. I was open to either feeling a bit better or being completely healthy. Either way, I felt this was better than focusing on being sick.

I then decided that if I was to get insights from my body, I needed to connect to my emotions. I began to focus on my breath. I gave myself permission to feel my emotions and receive wisdom from them, rather than resist and push them away. I realized that in order to heal, I needed to feel.

It also occurred to me to place my hands on my back. At the time, I did this to give my body some support. Later, I realized that, by touching my back, I was focusing my mind and energy toward healing that area. In other words, the intention of healing that began in my brain was now moving through my spinal cord and nervous system into my lower back.

I began to feel that my body was finally cooperating; I could feel it soften and relax. The "stuckness" that the chiropractor mentioned began to dissipate. But even though I was starting to feel better from time to time, doubts would still creep in— annoying thoughts like *It's not going to work, so don't bother* or *Nothing's worked before, so what makes you think this will?* I decided the best thing I could do was focus my mind and make it busy by counting backward from thirty.

This soothed my mind, and I realized that I did not have to make this healing happen; I needed to allow it to flow. I had heard about Divine Intelligence but could not really comprehend what it meant. I knew that my body was intelligent, as it knew how to make my blood flow, my hair grow, and my heart beat without me consciously doing anything. I decided to ask that if there was a thing such as Divine Healing

Intelligence, I wanted this intelligence to help me. Within moments, I felt a connection to an incredible healing energy. It was like a warm shimmering sun was melting all the rigidity and pain in my back.

When I turned my attention toward my spine, I saw the image of a disfigured back. Many vertebrae looked out of place and inflamed. Shocked, I thought, *I don't like this dream.* Then it hit me. I wasn't dreaming; I was looking at an image of my own back.

After my initial shock, I began wondering how my back could get to the condition it was in. So I asked the question, *What are the thoughts, emotions, and experiences that contributed to this condition?* I then waited while taking slow, deep breaths. Almost instantly, intense emotions of fear, frustration, anger, guilt, and shame began to surface. I kept breathing and feeling them, even when the emotions became extremely intense. I allowed myself to feel the intensity, repeating to myself, *I am willing to let these feelings go.*

Waves of emotions moved through my system. As I released them, I felt a calmness and connection to an incredible healing energy, and I received an insight or a memory related to each emotion. The more I released, the more Divine Spiritual Love I felt. In my mind's eye, I could see dense energy releasing from my body like puffs of smoke. I then fell into a deep and restful sleep.

The next morning, most of my pain was gone. I was so excited; I decided to experiment with this healing as much as I could. Within three weeks, the physical suffering had completely gone. At a checkup six months later, my amazed chiropractor said, "Whatever you are doing, keep doing it, because it works." After my back pain had released, I successfully worked on healing my skin, digestive problems, and anxiety.

## Helping Others Heal

People began to ask me to help them heal. Though I had healed myself, I was skeptical about my ability to help others. I noticed that after practicing tuning in to my body, my ability to tune into others' bodies and energy systems increased dramatically. Sometimes, without even asking, I would receive amazing, unexpected—and what I felt to be Divine—information, which was consistently confirmed when I shared it with others.

Initially, I tried to help my family. My mum was the most supportive of my newly discovered abilities. She told me that she believed in me completely and that healing was the path I needed to take. My dad was skeptical, but because he loves me deeply, he offered his support. My grandparents told me that my new career was one they had never heard of. My husband, Paul, was incredibly supportive and offered me some very sound advice: I should never make things up, and I should be sure that what I was saying was real and helpful to the people I was working with. He also said, "Unless it works, don't do it!" and I have stuck to that. I continue to learn from the people I work with, and I pay close attention to what works best for them. I don't get stuck in habits or cling to ideas or techniques that are no longer relevant.

One day, not long after I healed myself, my mum called and asked me to do a distance healing on my father, who had injured his leg at work. I turned my attention to him and, by "tuning in" in this way, saw he had badly bruised his leg. I was shown that he had, in fact, injured his leg on a boat. I told my mother, but she insisted that the accident had occurred at work. When I called my dad, however, he confirmed what I had seen. His leg healed very quickly.

I understand now that distance is no barrier to healing. This has allowed me to engage in healing work with people from around the world, tuning in to the mental, emotional, physical, and energetic causes of their disorders and life challenges. I realize that I am helping people connect to their own Divine Intelligence, an intelligence which enable them to heal.

Not long after my father's healing experience, a friend came to visit. As she was talking, an image of a cartoon-like liver appeared above her head. At first, I thought I must be going crazy and started closing and opening my eyes, waiting for the image to vanish. The image remained. I asked if she had a problem with her liver, and she replied that she had had a liver problem for most of her life.

I then saw an image of her grandfather in a concentration camp and was informed that he had had a similar problem. I relayed to my friend many more personal details about her health and her grandfather that she did not know. A few days later, she called to tell me her mother had confirmed all the details I had given about her grandfather. She has since told me that everything I shared with her about her health that day was later confirmed by medical tests and other health practitioners.

Over the next few months, I experimented with everyone who was willing, and the results astounded me. I gained confidence in the value of the healing work I was doing. At every available moment, I studied different healing methods and discovered how to use my abilities more effectively. I also began to interview and learn from bestselling authors in the area of spirituality, health, and human potential. My articles were published in newspapers and magazines around the world. However, I decided that the most empowering thing I could do was teach people to heal themselves. Thus, my deepest, most beneficial learning has come from clients in my private practice and from those who have participated in my workshops.

The information in this book comes from my years of studying the human body, working with clients one-on-one, and teaching workshops around the world. Every client has contributed to my understanding of the messages each part of the body has to give us and how we can use this information for self-healing.

Someone once asked me what kind of book I had written. I thought for a moment and replied, "I have written a book I would like to use." I have used the information in this book as a resource many, many times to demonstrate and explain how our thoughts and emotions affect our bodies. I hope you use *The Secret Language of Your Body* regularly to assist you in your own self-healing.

## Healing and Spirituality—Accessible to All

When people first meet me, they sometimes assume that my life is perfect—that I have no challenges and that I never get upset, concerned, or angry. They often try to put me on a pedestal and shower me with praise until they realize that I am simply human. I have doubts. I make occasional mistakes. I love fashion, going out dancing, watching movies, and listening to pop music.

In other words, I may have a deeply spiritual practice, but I also enjoy celebrating my life with a lot of normal pleasures. I try to demonstrate that you can be down to earth and also committed to your well-being, spirituality, and living a successful life. And people like it. At my seminars, people tell me they like my clothes, my youthful appearance, and the music I play—in fact, they say I make spiritual work look "cool." As a birthday present one year, Paul, along with music producer Phillip Gelbach, produced an album called *Right Now*, in which my vocals overlap inspiring, trance, dance, and chill-out music. People love dancing to it in my workshops. At one presentation, a lady came with her young niece, who was apparently expecting that someone doing spiritual healing would be older and frumpy. She was astonished that I looked young and was completely sold on me when she saw my shoes.

## How to Use This Book

This book is a reference guide that can help you understand how your feelings, experiences, energy, and thoughts influence your physical, mental, and emotional health. It may be crossed-referenced several different ways, depending on how you want to focus on a condition or remedy. If you are not well, look up your condition or the part or system of the body where you are experiencing difficulties in order to gain an understanding of the thoughts and emotions involved. Here are some ways the information may be accessed:

- **By ailment:** In part II, look for your condition in the alphabetized list. When you are reading about the disease, be aware of the emotions you are connecting to. Then turn to part III, the section on emotions, and do the relevant process.

- **By body part:** Every ailment will be stored in a part of your body. Look in part I to read about the relevant body part and then do the process described. You will also find information on related emotions, which you can further study by turning to part III.

- **By color:** In part IV, you can discover the qualities specific colors contain, which may assist you in restoring your body to vibrant health. You can also see how different colors affect you emotionally. Combine color healing with a process from the relevant body part or emotion section.

- **By body system:** I have found that addressing different but related parts of the body creates powerful results. If you are not sure which parts of the body make up a system, familiarize yourself with part V of the book, "The Secret Language of Your Body Systems." Then do the work on the parts of the body that are connected to that particular system, including the color visualizations.

You may also decide to combine processes when the problem you are dealing with is in several parts of the body. For example, if you have a throat cold and you would like to release it, read about "Colds" in part II. Then go to the section on body parts in part I and do the process for the throat. You may also combine the throat process with the process for the lungs and the chest. If you relate to certain emotions, you may do the emotional release process. During the day, you may be busy at work and decide to simply use a color, like orange. You may visualize orange moving into your chest, or rub your hands together and then imagine that you have a ball of orange light in between your hands. Place your hands on your throat or lungs, and breathe the orange light in, allowing it to regenerate these areas.

Remember that it is not enough to just read the processes; you need to practice them several times to really gain the benefits.

## Important Note

The healing exercises are not a replacement for a healthy diet, exercise plan, or appropriate healthcare, but they provide additional support to allow your body to become healthier, more vibrant, and more energetic. If you have a medical condition or a serious illness and are taking medication, please continue your treatment under medical supervision.

Even if you are on medication, you can still participate in your own healing by using the information and processes in this book. As you avail yourself of the treatments recommended by your healthcare providers, practice the exercises in this book and work on tuning in to yourself so that you continue to strengthen your connection to the Divine Healing Intelligence. As you feel that connection grow, let it take more of your attention; ignore scary statistics and other dire information that shake your confidence in your healing power. Keep in mind that there is a reason people speak of "healing miracles." Throughout history, people have found the key to their health, and some have accelerated their healing or changed the trajectory of an illness in ways that have baffled the medical community. Healing can take time, however, so be patient with yourself and make sure you have all the support you need. Only reduce your medication under the supervision of a medical practitioner.

## How to Work with Physical Problems

When I was writing this book, I realized that no matter what *dis-ease*, stress, condition, or illness you have, it is connected to a part of your body. Read the section on the different parts of your body and complete the remedy for healing. Do not underestimate the exercises just because they are simple; they have already worked for many, many people.

If you would like to improve the effectiveness of a remedy, combine it with another organ or part of the body that is connected to it. For example, if you have a cold, then work on your lungs, throat, and chest. If you relate strongly to a feeling, then turn to the section on emotions and do one of the processes to help you release dense, stressful emotions, such as feeling overwhelmed.

Another example would be if you have problems with your reproductive system, you would read the section on the systems of your body to understand the lessons you need to learn. Then work on the related organs and emotions. Or maybe if you have eye problems but have limited time to work on them, you may like to use color healing. Indigo and purple are fantastic for healing any illnesses or weaknesses that affect the eyes.

## How to Work with Emotional Problems

You may wake feeling stressed, depressed, or frustrated without experiencing any physical conditions. Go to the section on emotions in part III and do the process to release that emotion. Remember, it is important to do this process slowly and to breathe deeply. Visualize taking the negative emotions out of your body.

I have found that when people move their hands as they do this, it works even more powerfully. In my workshops, I usually play a song, which helps with releasing a particular emotion. Then I encourage people to move or shake their bodies to let go of that emotion, physically "taking" it out of their body with their hands and throwing it into an imaginary purple flame.

## How to Work with Color

Color healing is brilliant: you can do it anywhere, anytime, and it often works instantly. Color is also a vibration that you can actually feel in your hands, and different colors have different effects on the body.

Try this: rub your hands together, making sure that you rub each finger. Then hold your hands in front of you, slightly apart. You should begin to feel some tingling sensations. Now visualize that you are holding a big ball of red energy. You might feel some heat in your hands. If you have problems visualizing, just think *red*. Red contains unlimited energy, vitality, and power. Identify where your body feels tired and weak, then place your hands above that part of your body and "breathe in" red. Do this as if you are trying to drink it into your body. Now allow this red to expand in your body while taking slow, deep breaths. You should quickly feel revitalized. You can also move your hands around your body, making the red move throughout your whole body. Note: do not focus on the color red if the area is inflamed or if you have a headache.

Now try the same exercise with the color blue. Blue should feel very different in your hands. It is likely to feel lighter, cooler, and more expansive. Ask which part of your body needs some blue, and breathe blue into it as you hold your hands over that area. Blue is great for soothing your mind, creating peace, and working with your nervous system. Similarly, indigo is one of the best colors for pain relief. Just place your hands above the part of your body where you are feeling pain, and breathe in the indigo color. Allow it to move through your body to dissolve any pain and density.

After leading an event in London, a woman came up to me beaming with excitement after we had done the color healing exercise. Almost out of breath with enthusiasm, she showed me her hands. "Look!" she exclaimed. I just stared at her while she wiggled her fingers in front of me wildly. Seeing my confusion, her friend explained that Lucy had suffered from arthritis and had not been able to move her fingers for two years. Recovering her composure, Lucy told me that after rubbing her hands and imagining the red light, her fingers became really hot, to the point of pain. She breathed very slowly to avoid making a sound. Then, while working with the color blue, she felt her fingers cool. Within a minute, her hands were relaxed, and, for the first time in years, she was able to move them freely.

When you read about a particular color, experiment with it by rubbing your hands together, visualizing the color, feeling it, and directing it into a part of your body.

## How to Work with Body Systems

The systems of your body give you an insight into all the organs, glands, and other parts that make up a particular area. Since everything in the body is interconnected, it is useful to work with different parts of the body together. For example, let's say you have a problem with your hormones. Go to part V, look up the endocrine system, and you will see that this system consists of the hypothalamus, pituitary, pineal, thyroid, parathyroid, thymus, adrenal glands, ovaries, testes, and pancreas. Depending on your particular condition, you would go to the body parts section of the book and work with some of the glands and organs described above. I have also included the causes of system breakdowns and the wisdom each body system offers.

## If You Are Well

You do not have to be ill to benefit from the information in this book. You can use the healing processes to further enhance your health, well-being, intuition, and success. You can work on clearing your nervous system, for example, allowing you to feel more balanced and peaceful. You can also work with the emotions of love, joy, and happiness, or improve your immune system by working on your pituitary gland and hormones. I also encourage you to read the section about fingers and toes. Each of your fingers and toes is connected to various organs and energies in your body. By working on them, you improve your overall health and well-being.

The most important thing of all is to enjoy the experience. The more interesting, joyful, and fun you make it, the faster you will feel great.

Healing can occur quickly or take time. Be patient and repeat the processes regularly. Even though many people thought that I did not need more healing after my pain released, I recognized that it was only the beginning of my journey of discovery. I use these processes daily to feel healthier, happier, more abundant, and more confident.

Sometimes, even the smallest change can make a huge difference and place you on the path of wellness. Imagine being in a really bad mood; you feel a headache coming on, and plan to take an aspirin and go to bed, but a friend calls and invites you to go out. Reluctantly, you leave your house. You see the most beautiful sunset, take a few really deep breaths, and begin to relax. Then a stranger walks by and makes a kind comment. Suddenly, you begin to feel better and your headache disappears. You meet your friend in better spirits and have a great night. The next day, you awake feeling fabulous as you think about the great night you had. You decide that life is wonderful and have another enjoyable day.

This simple example shows your mind's ability to influence your body. If you are around someone who is negative and constantly criticizes or judges you, you are going to feel upset, angry, and fearful. Those emotions will cause your body to tighten, your immune system to weaken, and your nervous system to come under stress and attack. If you don't let go of the negative feelings, your body will start to break down, and you will get sick.

Psychoneuroimmunology (PNI) research shows that negative thoughts, beliefs, attitudes, and emotions weaken the nervous and immune systems and lead to disease. In 2001, Dr. Margo de Kooker, a medical doctor who specializes in the field of behavioral medicine, wrote a scientific overview for The Wellness Support Programme:

> *In the real world, what the field of PNI proves is that what happens in our minds at the level of our perception ... can have real effects on ... our immune system. This concept is not new, and the ancient wisdom has always encouraged us to focus on*

*maintaining a "healthy" mind in order to maintain a healthy body. It is only now that we are able to prove and understand the connections.*

On a physical level, the body is constantly changing. Science has established that our skin is renewed every month, stomach lining cells change every three days, eye cells every forty-eight hours, liver cells every six weeks, and skeleton cells every three months.

The exciting thing is that by consciously participating in your own healing process, you assist your body to regenerate faster, without the density, toxicity, and blockages that stop you from being vibrantly well. Imagine: You decide that you are ready to see clearly and spend two days working on your eyesight, knowing that cells of your eyes regenerate every forty-eight hours. After two days, you can see perfectly.

I have had astonishing feedback from people who have successfully used my processes to heal diabetes, cysts, arthritis, back pain, knee problems, heart palpitations, kidney problems, bladder cancer, migraines, skin conditions of all kinds, cystitis, hemorrhoids, eye problems, depression, anxiety, and many other ailments.

If you use this book on a regular basis, you will not only help your body to heal, you will also change your life and release the density and negativity that keep you limited, stuck, and fearful. The changes you experience may be obvious from the start, or they may be almost imperceptible. As you continue using the processes contained in this book, you will realize just how much you have transformed.

I have included a process for tuning in to your body that is similar to the one I used to heal myself. Practice this process to receive deeper insights into your challenges, and then work toward healing. This process can be used in conjunction with the other processes in this book or on its own.

## Exercise for Tuning In to Your Body

1. Find a comfortable place to sit or lie down.

2. Count backward from thirty as you take deep breaths and allow your mind and body to relax.

3. Focus on an area in your body that feels blocked or an area where you have pain.

4. Breathe the color green into the area for a few moments and place your hands there.

5. Ask your body, "Is there a message you want to give me?" This message may come in a form of thoughts, words, images, insights, feelings, memories, and so forth.

6. Take a few deep breaths as you allow any messages to come to the surface. Do not judge any message.

7. Write down the messages.

8. Say: "I call on my Divine Healing Intelligence to help release all pain, blockages, and density from this area." Allow yourself to watch and feel the dense energy leave your body.

9. Breathe deeply and slowly, arching your head back slightly and curving your lower spine. Then, as you breathe out, bring your head forward, and allow your back to straighten. Do this in a relaxed and easy manner.

10. Do the color healing exercise described on page XXX using the color indigo for pain relief.

11. Say: "I call on my Divine Healing Intelligence to infuse this area with healing energy. I allow all the immune mechanisms of my body to activate and my body to return to a state of perfect balance and health."

12. Breathe in continuously for one minute, allowing the energy to build.

13. Imagine a warm, golden light moving through your whole body and repairing it.

14. When you feel lighter, gently bring your awareness back to normal, and open your eyes knowing that you have activated your own Divine Healing Intelligence.

You can do this exercise daily to either focus on specific health challenges or to improve or maintain the health of your whole body. You may also decide to use the processes as a preventative measure or to feel more empowered, confident, and healthy.

To assist you even further, I have created a free audio download of the above process that is a helpful tool to use together with this. See the back of the book for information on how to access the audio download and for other related materials. You can also access my website for additional information and more materials for different aspects of healing at www.InnaSegal.com.

When you engage in the processes, it is important to be relaxed and take deep breaths. This allows you to help the body feel and release tension and stuckness. In healing, your imagination can be your biggest asset and your mind a faithful servant. If you use both correctly, the results will speak for themselves. Know one thing: Well-being is your Divine Right, and it is available to you at all times if you allow it into your life. Your biggest challenge is fear and resistance but the information in this book can help you overcome it.

If you are still skeptical, you can succeed by taking one step at a time. If you discover that one process does not seem to work for you as well as you would like, try another. Be creative and adjust the processes so that you feel like they were created for you.

My prayer is that you experience great improvement in your health and well-being, as well as in every other area of your life. Please immerse yourself in this book, and begin to discover the secret language of your body.

love
Inna

# I

# THE SECRET LANGUAGE OF YOUR BODY

## Healing the Emotional, Mental, and Energetic Causes of Disease

In the following section, you will find information about your organs and the possible symptoms of related disorders. Please use the information in this and other sections as a guide to assist you in finding your own insights into your health.

After reading about each body part, tune into your body and become aware of which symptoms you relate to. Then, do the healing process. You may also decide to do an emotional release process in Part III, "The Secret Language of Your Emotions."

In each exercise, you are asked to relax your body, as relaxation is the optimal state for healing. Deep breathing can also help you focus on the area you are working with in order to feel the stuckness. To heal, you must be willing to feel. As you recognize what is keeping you stuck, the density, tension, and stress will begin to dissolve and a new sense of awareness, empowerment, and well-being will take its place.

Every person has the ability to visualize. Think about your bedroom. What furniture do you have? What color is the room? What is your favorite piece of clothing? What color is it? In order to answer those questions, you had to create pictures in your mind. You may argue that you did not see those images clearly; you just have a sense of them. This is perfectly fine. The images don't have to be clear for you to benefit from visualizing; it is your intention that counts. If you are asked to imagine the color blue and you cannot visualize it clearly, do not be discouraged. If your intention is to use its healing properties, you will still receive the benefits. The more you practice, the clearer the images will become. Be patient.

Visualizing, however, is different from tuning in. When I refer to "tuning in" to an area of your body, I am talking about placing your attention on an area, breathing into it, and sensing what is going on there. Some people will receive still images or moving pictures, and those impressions might be clear or blurry. You might be seeing the current state of your organ or remembering an incident that occurred to you many years ago. You may not receive an image but instead become aware of a strong feeling, an unusual thought, or a word that is going round and round in your head.

A sign or an answer to your question may occur at the time that you are tuning in or a bit later. You might smell something that reminds you of a person or event, or taste something strange in your mouth. Whether an image, moving picture, feeling, thought, sound, smell, or taste, do not judge what you receive. Work with the information however it is provided. Everything you receive is important and is a piece of the puzzle toward your healing.

## Using Divine Healing Intelligence to Heal Your Body

Throughout many of the processes, I use the words "Divine Healing Intelligence." I believe that your body has a Divine Intelligence that makes your heart beat, your blood flow, and your hair grow without you doing anything consciously. If you cut your hand, this same Intelligence will heal the wound. By asking the part of you that already knows how to heal, the healing can happen more quickly and effectively. Some people may refer to this as your subconscious mind, but I believe that we are all spiritual beings with a higher intelligence, which works through us. This Intelligence can work through our subconscious mind as well as our conscious awareness.

As part of the processes for healing offered in the following sections, I also encourage you to release "all points of view." I have found that many of us have beliefs that limit us from healing and expanding. Some people may have a point of view that they think is positive only to discover that this outlook keeps them stuck in a pattern. For example, a person might believe that marriage to a person of similar religious belief is a positive point of view. However, if a child falls in love with someone of a different faith, this point of view can create conflict between the parents and their child. If they get stuck on this point of view, the relationship with their child might be harmed, potentially causing much unnecessary pain and suffering. In fact, a couple's stuck point of view can actually cause their child to rebel and to draw closer to the person who may or may not be for their highest good. So, we want to release all points of view and allow ourselves to create space to connect to the Divine or most empowering point of view.

Another part of the healing statement is to release positive and negative charges. When we have a charge on someone or something, we often react strongly to that person, event, or experience. A negative charge could be based on a strong negative feeling like anger, hate, fear, jealousy, and so on. A positive charge could be based on a strong need, expectation, feeling of impatience, and so on.

For instance, you may have just gotten a new job and feel over the moon about it. You may have ideas and expectations about what you are going to do and learn in this new job. Then you discover that the reality at work is very different from what you had hoped. Thus, you become frustrated and depressed, and the positive charge turns negative. Ideally, we want to release all charges and allow Divinity, synchronicity, and well-being to flow into our lives.

To help with this, my healing processes are always followed by the word "CLEAR," as a reminder to clear all density, pain, stress, and limitation out of your mind, body, emotions, and vibration. When you repeat the word "CLEAR," imagine a broom or a vacuum cleaner clearing any mess out of your system, or clearing a pathway for you to experience wonderful things in your life. Repeat the word several times until you can tell something has cleared, indicated by your feeling lighter, more at ease, freer, tingly, or more open to new possibilities.

I have also discovered that when you repeat the word "CLEAR" often, taking a moment to visualize until you feel the clutter disappear, you will start having more clarity in your life, your memory will improve, and you will able to manifest more of the things you desire. Your body will also work better because each time you say "CLEAR," your nervous system will begin to clear any stuckness you have, improving the communication between your mind and body. Some people see results from these exercises immediately, but if you do not, remember that just as it can take time for disease to develop, sometimes it also takes time to find health and wellness again.

Your hands are also wonderful helpers in healing. In several of the exercises, you are encouraged to place your hands on different body parts, imagining a color coming through them. Each color has an energy vibration which can assist different organs to heal and regenerate.

You will also find that in many of the processes, I urge you to ask yourself questions in order to discover how you are feeling and what actions you can take to change your life. Those questions are extremely important to your health, well-being, and inner fulfillment, as your life experience depends on the quality of the questions you are willing to ask. If you ask disempowering questions such as "Why isn't it working?" or "Why do I always fail?" or "Why do bad things happen to me?" then the results will always be negative. However, if you ask empowering questions such as "How can I do this?" or "How can I succeed?" or "What are the possibilities of finding a way to heal myself within a short time?" you will find the universe will help you heal, succeed, and achieve your goals more quickly and easily.

## What You Will Gain with Your Healing Practice

You have the opportunity to work with thoughts, words, feelings, beliefs, vibrations, touch, movement, visualization, and breath to create changes in your body and in your life. Remember, pain and discomfort is your body's way of communicating that you need to make changes. The more you are in tune with your body, the easier, more joyful, and more rewarding your life will be. You have the opportunity to tune into your own Divine Wisdom and receive all the guidance you require. This guidance is not only relevant to your health but to your relationships, your career, your mental and emotional well-being, and your spiritual expansion.

For optimal results, I suggest you do these exercises daily. At times, you will need to repeat the same exercise several times a day for a week or longer; other times, the symptoms will disappear in a few hours.

As mentioned earlier, when you are feeling well, you can do a quick healing process to feel even better. I have found that many people wait until they are sick to begin looking after themselves. I often hear that when people feel well, they simply stop doing anything that makes them expand and grow until they feel stuck, sick, or unhappy again. Imagine how much more pleasant your life would be if you felt better and better each day.

Many people begin a healing program and then quit because they don't see instant results. They convince themselves that it's too hard, it's not going to work, or there is not enough time. If you have felt this in the past, then you need to let go of those beliefs and start affirming and welcoming great health and success into your life.

## Taking Responsibility

To experience incredible healing, you need to make a commitment to succeed and take responsibility for your actions. Responsibility does not mean blaming yourself for feeling unwell; on the contrary, it means discovering what choices or decisions you made that did not work. You can decide to do things differently and find out what would make your life and health brilliant.

Laura, a woman in her sixties, contacted me because she could not sleep, had terrible coughing fits and asthma, suffered from arthritis and back pain, and could barely walk. She had consulted a physical therapist, a psychologist, several doctors, chiropractors, and other practitioners with little improvement. I helped Laura create a healing program for all these conditions by working through emotions that had been keeping her stuck.

First, I discovered that, ten years earlier, Laura received a huge shock when she was accused of cheating. From that moment, her health began to deteriorate. We started the healing process by working with her emotions of anger, sadness, depression, and resentment. Laura also spent time forgiving the people involved. Immediately, she felt freer, and her back pain eased.

I taught Laura a process to help her release the negative thoughts and dense feelings she was carrying and create positive thoughts and feelings in their place. Then I shared processes with Laura for healing chest, back, joint, and leg problems.

Laura did the processes daily. Every time I spoke with her, she reported improvement. She was extremely excited to share with me the night she was able to release her asthma and enjoy a restful sleep. She stopped coughing after only a few days of self-healing. Within a few months, Laura was walking with very little effort, experiencing more flexibility in her body and more happiness in her life.

When Laura was able to take responsibility and understand what her body was trying to tell her, she changed her life and healed. Rather than being a victim of her circumstances, she became empowered and reclaimed her well-being.

Are you ready to take responsibility for your health and well-being? Are you willing to make your healing a priority? If you answered yes, then you are ready to begin. I can't wait to hear about your successes!

Please email your results to me so that I can share them and inspire others to reclaim their wellness. If you need extra support, check the back of the book for access to further tools that can help you to become more vibrantly well, joyful, and successful in all areas of life.

## Ten Basic Principles for Healing

"Healing" means wholeness. Thus, in order to heal on all levels, we must consider all aspects that make great health possible.

### Principle 1

Commit to making your health a priority. This means believing you are a valuable being, who deserves brilliant health and well-being. Making your health a priority also gives you the opportunity to examine your thinking. Are you open-minded and willing to explore the root causes of your dis-ease or discomfort, and to work on releasing the negativity which may have contributed to your condition? Or is your definition of healing taking a pill and perhaps shutting down your body?

True healing means listening to the messages your body is trying to give you and then making changes, which creates ease and flow—rather than dis-ease and stuckness—in your body and your life.

## Principle 2

Feel your emotions instead of keeping them buried. Many people spend much of their time thinking rather than feeling because they find the experience of "feeling" uncomfortable. When unwelcome feelings come up, they try to shut them down by being distracted, watching television, eating junk food, talking on the phone, reading a book, listening to music, smoking, taking drugs, and so forth. However, your feelings hold the key to your well-being. They tell you what is honoring you and what is not; if your life is flowing the way it's meant to; and if you are moving in the wrong direction.

Your feelings give you the opportunity to expand, release pain, achieve your ideal weight, create change, and break down the armor that prevents you from experiencing health, peace, and joy.

## Principle 3

Breathe consciously. Many people breathe shallowly, thus keeping the body tight, stagnant, and working harder. When you breathe slowly, deeply, and consciously, you feel your body, tune into your intuition, relax your mind, and purify the blood. You also experience an increase in energy and well-being as the breath circulates energy around your body.

## Principle 4

Eat healthfully and consciously. Most people know what constitutes a healthy diet. Yet, in our stressed and busy lives, it is easy to go for fast food, which usually contains lots of fat, sugar, caffeine, and unhealthy chemicals. Often, people eat quickly and on the go without being aware of what they are eating, or truly tasting and enjoying their food. This leads them to eat more than their body requires.

Being healthy means eating healthy food that nourishes your body and gives you energy, vitality, and well-being. Taking time to create healthy food, which you eat slowly and chew consciously, gives your body the opportunity to heal and regenerate quickly and easily.

## *Principle 5*

Move your body. Many people complain about feeling stagnant, depressed, uninspired, and overweight. However, each person has the ability to create an exercise program, which creates and maintains a desired weight, and helps one become strong, healthy, lean, and fit. Regular exercise can help you to feel better about yourself, to enjoy your body, to have more energy, to detoxify, and to heal. Plan an exercise program you will enjoy, such as walking, swimming, going to the gym, dancing, yoga, martial arts, tai chi, and so on.

## *Principle 6*

Listen to your body. Recognize when you need to rest, play, have fun, and work. What are your cycles? When are you at your best? What can you do to make your life more productive? It is when people don't listen to their bodies that stress, tension, fear, frustration, anxiety, and dis-ease set in. Take a break for a few minutes every couple of hours. Stretching, deep breathing, or even a short meditation can make the difference between feeling tired, stagnant, and stressed or feeling healthy, creative, and relaxed.

## *Principle 7*

Be creative. Creativity allows you to relax, have fun, and explore. It gives you opportunities to learn, expand, and discover your talents. When people are creative, they are often more inspired, imaginative, and resourceful. Fun and creativity prolong your life, so find activities you can participate in to express yourself creatively.

## Principle 8

Add more color to your life. Colors can make people feel heavy, depressed, and fatigued or light, vibrant, and joyful. Become aware of the colors that make you feel great and the qualities they have, and then add these colors to your life. This could mean painting your walls green because green makes you feel relaxed and tranquil, wearing a bright orange dress or shirt to feel vibrant, or bringing more flowers into your home for added renewal during the winter months. Whatever it is, make it colorful.

## Principle 9

Make gratitude your attitude. Focus on all the great things you have in your life instead of thinking about what you don't have, complaining about your lack and limitation. Remember, what you focus on grows; if you choose to focus on what you are unhappy about, it will multiply.

## Principle 10

Make laughter a priority. For a long time, people believed that they needed a reason to laugh. However, the benefits of laughter are so great that laughing for laughter's sake has become the motto for countless people all over the world who participate in "laughter clubs." There is even laughter yoga, which teaches specific laughter exercises. Looking at life from a humorous angle allows you to let go of stress and heal faster.

## A Guide to Physical Disorders and Suggestions for Healing

During my Visionary Intuitive Healing workshops and while conducting healing treatments, I came to the realization that every part of the body stores particular emotions, thoughts, memories, energy, and experiences based on the function of that part of the body. For example, the role of an eye is to see, so if there is a problem with your eye, it is likely to be connected to something you don't want to see in your life.

This section is designed to heighten your awareness of the different factors that could contribute to a problem or a disease in a part of your body. When you can recognize the blocks, issues, and limitations, you can start to release them. The processes are designed to use many elements: thoughts, feelings, breath, acupressure, exercises, visualization, movement, questions, and all five of your senses. To help with the visualizations of internal organs or other body parts that may not be familiar to you, refer to the illustrations in the index (pages 243 and 244) that show the parts of the body.

At the end of each exercise are suggestions for emotions and colors that may be useful to work with in order to speed up your healing. Refer to part III and work on the heaviest emotions first. Then work with the positive emotion you would like to experience more of. If there is another emotion you relate to that is not mentioned, then work with the general emotional process in that exercise.

Remember to use the information in this section as a guideline. Not every possible contributing factor listed will relate to you, so tune into your body to receive your own answers. Even the healthy thoughts and emotions are written as suggestions. Though I often word the exercises so they will be accessible to readers who are learning to replace stuck emotions with health-promoting ones for the first time, people at any stage of their exploration of these thoughts and emotions can apply these exercises to their healing. So, use these instructions as a starting point but adjust the processes to make them more powerful for yourself.

## *Abdomen*

### Possible Contributing Factors

Difficulty digesting life. Propensity to hold on to toxic feelings, thoughts, and hurts from the past. Constant fear and worry about the future, which creates struggle and suffering in the present. Frequent feelings of insecurity and confusion about what to do and what choices to make. Deep-seated belief of not being good enough. Fear of rejection and failure. Wanting to be the center of attention but afraid of being judged.

## Remedy

Take a deep breath in through your nose and slowly breathe out from your mouth. Relax and soften your abdomen as much as possible. If you experience pain in your abdomen, imagine that you have a vacuum cleaner in your hands. Visualize vacuuming all the density, toxicity, and pain out of your abdomen.

Say: "Divine Healing Intelligence, I ask you to release all toxic thoughts and feelings, old painful experiences, stuckness, struggle, and rejection out of my abdomen, as well as all points of view, all patterns, and the positive and negative charges that contribute to this condition." Repeat the word "CLEAR" until you feel a shift occur.

Rub your hands together until they become warm and tingly. Then place your hands on your abdomen.

Say: "Divine Healing Intelligence, please install feelings and experiences of ease, relaxation, and freedom. I now invite healing, loving, and empowering energy into my life. Thank you."

Allow your body to take in the energy of wellness from your Divine Healing Intelligence and your hands. Now imagine how it would feel to be completely healthy, confident, and secure. How would you think? How would you feel? What would your life experience be like? What would your posture be like? How would others respond to you? Allow yourself to see it, feel it, and experience it.

When you have done this, go outside and find a stone. Hold that stone and repeat the previous visualization process in which you saw yourself becoming healthier and more confident. This time make the process even stronger. Carry this stone with you for the next month. Squeeze it any time you need extra confidence or a boost of healing energy.

Say: "Divine Healing Intelligence, please heal and regenerate my abdomen and all related organs to their full health and vitality. Thank you."

Unhealthy emotions to work with (page 171): Fear 179, Frustration 181, Rejection 191

Healthy emotions to work with (page 197): Peace 204, Relaxation 205, Freedom 201
Colors to work with (page 211): Yellow 221, Orange 216

## Adrenal Glands

### Possible Contributing Factors

Lack of energy or fatigue. Feeling emotionally unbalanced and unstable—one moment, happy and content; and the next, sad and hopeless. Frequent bouts of paranoia, panic attacks, fear, and anxiety, often related to a feeling that you have taken the wrong direction in life. Difficulty making decisions. Feeling stuck in the fight-or-flight response. In some cases, feelings of depression, emptiness, worthlessness, and exhaustion.

### Remedy

Take a deep breath in through your nose and slowly exhale through your mouth. Do this three times. Then take a deep breath in and focus on energizing the adrenal glands. Imagine your adrenal glands being filled with vibrant green energy. As you breathe out, focus on letting go of any density, fear, and stress. This may look like grayness and density coming out of your glands. Do this five to eight times.

Say: "Divine Healing Intelligence, I ask you to release all fear, anxiety, hopelessness, exhaustion, fatigue, stress, and stuckness out of my adrenal glands, as well as all points of view, the positive and negative charges, and all limiting patterns that contribute to this condition." Repeat the word "CLEAR" until you feel a shift occur.

Say: "Divine Healing Intelligence, please install feelings and experiences of energy, movement, peace, and trust. Thank you."

Focus on your hands; imagine that you are holding orange balls of energy. Touch your adrenal glands and allow those orange balls to penetrate the glands. Begin clearing any density that remains, releasing any stories and memories of past experiences; letting go of exhaustion and worn-out feelings; and balancing the hormones, water, and stress response in your body. Feel the vibrant energy return to your life, and focus on moving in the right direction. Ask questions like, "How can I begin moving in the direction of my highest good? How can I connect to my Divine Guidance System?"

Then allow the response to come into your life. You may receive this response through inspiration, a book, an experience, or some other way. Be patient and allowing.

Say: "Divine Healing Intelligence, please heal and regenerate my adrenal glands and all related organs to their full health and vitality. Thank you."

Unhealthy emotions to work with (page 171): Sadness 193, Hopelessness 186, Stuckness 196, Depression 176
Healthy emotions to work with (page 197): Happiness 201, Freedom 201, Clarity 197
Colors to work with (page 211): Orange 216, Green 213

## Ankles

### Possible Contributing Factors
Feeling weighed down by too much responsibility. Overcommitting yourself and then feeling like you have chains around your ankles. Feeling trapped in a destructive relationship, friendship, job, or situation that you don't know how to leave. Thinking that you have no choice. Inability to trust, step forward, and embrace your dreams for fear of making mistakes. Wanting to be right. Feeling off balance and not knowing what step to take next.

### *Right Ankle*
Being challenged by a male authority figure. Following in your father's footsteps. Giving away your power or ideas to another person, such as a lover, supervisor, or father figure. Having too many responsibilities. Trying to please others first. Inability to say no or to stand up for yourself.

### *Left Ankle*
Difficulty tuning in to yourself and listening to your own counsel. Belief that you have to be a slave to others, especially to your children, your partner, or your work. Not spending enough time nurturing yourself and discovering what is important to you.

## Remedy

Focus on your ankles. Inhale and exhale deeply, allowing the breath to move through your entire body. How do your ankles feel? Do they feel tight, stiff, or painful? What is weighing you down or holding you back?

Tighten your ankles and then relax them. Spend a few moments massaging them until they feel more relaxed. Become aware if you are carrying energetic or emotional chains around your ankles. If you are, allow yourself to remove them. You can do this by closing your eyes, sensing or seeing the chains, and then taking them off with your hands and placing them into a purple fire.

Say: "Divine Healing Intelligence, I ask you to dissolve all mental, emotional, or energetic chains from my ankles. Please release all weakness, confusion, and disorder from my life, as well as all points of view, all patterns, and the positive and negative charges that contribute to this condition." Repeat the word "CLEAR" until you feel a shift occur.

Say: "Divine Healing Intelligence, please install feelings and experiences of empowerment, strength, order, and self-esteem. I now choose to walk on my path with self-belief, assurance, and clarity. Thank you."

Visualize taking clear, deliberate, confident steps ahead. Now stand and take a few steps. Concentrate on walking toward your desires. How does it feel to walk forward without the heavy chains? What are the possibilities that lie ahead of you now? Embrace the positive possibilities. Tell yourself that you can see and feel yourself creating the life you will love. Breathe in feelings of joy and happiness about this decision.

Say: "Divine Healing Intelligence, please heal and regenerate my ankles and all related organs to their full health and vitality. Thank you."

Unhealthy emotions to work with (page 171): Stuckness 196, Fear 179, Feeling Overwhelmed 180

Healthy emotions to work with (page 197): Compassion 198, Peace 204, Forgiveness 200

Colors to work with (page 211): Pink 217, Green 213

## *Anus*

### Possible Contributing Factors

Difficulty letting go of outdated family beliefs and fears. Feeling guilty, regretful, and uncomfortable with decisions that were made in the past. Holding on to anger toward yourself and others. Fear of loss and abandonment. Inability to forgive and learn from the past. Constant criticism of self and others. Feeling unhappy with yourself and your life. Feeling like no matter what you do, it's never enough. Trying to control life. Feeling betrayed, that what you thought was true may not be. Believing that you are not worthy of good things in life.

### Remedy

Place your attention on your anus. Inhale and exhale deeply. Allow the breath to move through your entire body. Focus on the process of letting go. When you pay for something, you let go of your money but receive something in return; when you move to another home, you let go of the old to welcome the new; and when you let go of pain, you welcome well-being into your life.

Slowly take a deep breath in and gently squeeze the muscles of your anus. When you exhale, relax them. As you squeeze, focus on the negative feeling or belief you are holding on to. When you relax, focus on letting them go.

Say: "Divine Healing Intelligence, I ask you to release all guilt, blame, criticism, anger, outdated fears, and stuckness out of my anus, as well as all points of view, all patterns, and the positive and negative charges that contribute to this condition." Repeat the word "CLEAR" until you feel a shift occur.

Rub your hands together. Place them slightly apart. Focus on the tingling sensation. Visualize orange light between your hands. Place your hands on your anus. Breathe in the orange rays and allow them to clear all toxicity out of your anus. You may feel internal tingling and adjustment. Keep breathing for a minute as this occurs.

Say: "Divine Healing Intelligence, please install feelings and experiences of wisdom, faith, and self-confidence. Thank you."

Give yourself permission to move forward and make empowering decisions that can bring happiness and well-being into your life.

Say: "Divine Healing Intelligence, please heal and regenerate my anus and all related organs to their full health and vitality. Thank you."

Unhealthy emotions to work with (page 171): Fear 179, Guilt 184, Anger 173
Healthy emotions to work with (page 197): Forgiveness 200, Freedom 201, Love 203
Colors to work with (page 211): Orange 216, Brown 212, Green 213

## Arms

### Possible Contributing Factors

Difficulty expressing yourself. Feeling stuck, powerless, and inflexible. Fear of change. Trying to do too much or too little. Holding back. Experiencing struggle and resistance. Missing out on wonderful new opportunities because of internal limitations and conflicts.

### Right Arm

Storing stress, pain, limitation, or anger from males in your life: father, brother, uncle, cousin, friend, lover, husband, son, or other. Feeling like you are controlled or too controlling with others. Perfectionism. Missing out on great opportunities by being too caught up in little problems.

### Left Arm

Holding on to pain, sadness, and fear from females in your life: mother, sister, daughter, friend, lover, boss, or other. Feeling like you are being taken advantage of and taken for granted. Feeling overwhelmed, like you want to push people away. Trying to help others by taking on their worries and problems, and then feeling heavy, tired, and discouraged because you can't solve other people's problems.

## Remedy

Focus on your arms. Start by gently shaking them, as if you are shaking out all the stress, fear, and negativity. Imagine that there is a trash bin in front of you and you are shaking all the density into the bin. Shake for about thirty seconds, then stop for fifteen seconds and feel the tingling sensation and a sense of relief. Repeat the shaking process three to five times until your arms feel lighter. If you can't shake them, gently massage them or ask someone to massage them for you, until your arms feel more relaxed.

Say: "Divine Healing Intelligence, I ask you to melt away all mental, emotional, or energetic stress, pain, anger, worry, manipulation, and control. Please release all fear, sadness, resistance, and inflexibility from my arms as well as all points of view, all patterns, and the positive and negative charges that contribute to this condition." Repeat the word "CLEAR" until you feel a shift occur.

Take some deep breaths, focusing on relaxing your arms, shoulders, hands, and fingers. Imagine that an orange stream of energy flows inside each arm. This stream moves up and down your arm looking for any pain, tension, density, or stagnation. When it finds it, the orange energy begins to heat up, dissipating any pain, density, or stagnation. The more you allow your arms to relax, the quicker the pain, density, and stagnation releases.

Once you have done this, imagine putting your arms into a bath of luscious, green energy. Feel this warm, vibrant energy regenerating your arms. Give yourself permission to become more creative and expressive in your life.

Say: "Divine Healing Intelligence, please install feelings and experiences of creativity, healthy self-expression, balance, strength, and courage."

Say: "Divine Healing Intelligence, please heal and regenerate my arms and all related organs to their maximum strength, vitality, and flexibility. Thank you."

Unhealthy emotions to work with (page 171): Stuckness 196, Fear 179, Control 174, Feeling Overwhelmed 180

Healthy emotions to work with (page 197): Confidence 198, Support 206, Freedom 201

Colors to work with (page 211): Orange 216, Pink 217, Green 213

## *Arteries*

### Possible Contributing Factors

Feeling disconnected from your heart. Buying into the negativity and limitations of others. Fear of loving others because of past hurts. Feeling shut down and uninspired by life. Pushing yourself too hard. Conflict at home or at work. Limiting your own self-expression and creativity. Feeling lack of nourishment and connection with the heart. Refusing to communicate. Blocking your connection to others. Feeling lost, powerless, listless. Ignoring your own intuition and desires. In some cases, feelings of self-hatred, fear, and blame.

### Remedy

Say: "Divine Healing Intelligence, I ask you to dissolve all blockages I may have to giving love. Please help me to dissolve all negativity, conflict, limitation, self-hatred, fear, and blame from my arteries, as well as all points of view, all patterns, and the positive and negative charges that contribute to this condition." Repeat the word "CLEAR" until you feel a shift occur.

Rub your hands together. Place your hands slightly apart. Visualize pink light in between your hands. Place your hands on your chest. Breathe in this pink light. Allow it to surround the arteries, soothing, softening, and healing them.

Say: "Divine Healing Intelligence, please install feelings and experiences of love, and a deep connection to my heart's wisdom. I am now open to learn to love myself and others, and I attract loving, joyful, respectful, and honoring relationships into my life. Thank you."

Say: "Divine Healing Intelligence, please heal and regenerate my arteries and all related organs to their full health and vitality. Thank you."

*See also* Heart.

Unhealthy emotions to work with (page 171): Fear 179, Hatred 185, Judgment 188
Healthy emotions to work with (page 197): Confidence 198, Love 203, Forgiveness 200
Colors to work with (page 211): Pink 217, Green 213, Mauve 215

## *Back*

### Possible Contributing Factors

Feeling unsupported, overwhelmed, and under too much pressure. Carrying suppressed and unresolved emotions from the past.

### *Upper Back*

Carrying the world on your shoulders. Feeling stressed and overwhelmed by all the things you have to do. Lack of trust, and frequent worry, fear, negativity, perfectionism, and limitation. Feeling unsupported by life and people around you. Too much thinking.

### *Middle Back*

Stuck in the past. Holding on to guilt and resentment. Difficulty breathing and taking in life. Emotional instability. Overly sensitive to other peoples' beliefs, thoughts, judgments, and criticisms. Difficulty forgiving yourself and others for past mistakes. Too focused on what's wrong instead of what's right.

### *Lower Back*

Feeling insecure about how you will support yourself financially. Constant worry about your survival and how you are going to pay the bills. Holding on to unresolved anger from childhood. Feeling like a victim. Struggling, suffering, controlling. Focused on limitations and negativity, and why you can't do things instead of how you can.

### Remedy

Focus on your back. Breathe deeply and slowly, arching your head back slightly and curving your lower spine. Then, as you breathe out, bring your head forward and allow your back to straighten. Repeat this process several times until your breathing feels steady and relaxed.

Become aware of which part of your back is holding on to dense energy and negativity. Place your hands on that part of your back. Breathe into this area three times. Ask your back if it has any messages for you. These could be thoughts, emotions, sensations, visual images, or memories. Give yourself time to recognize and receive the messages. You may even decide to write them down to become aware of how these energies, stories, and feelings are giving you pain.

Tighten your back and then relax. Do this five to eight times. Focus on taking slow, deep breaths in and out to release all your stress and tension. Become aware of any heavy load that you are carrying on your back. This load could be the responsibilities you have in your life, the worries and stresses you have accumulated, or anger and fear. You may also feel that you have been stabbed in the back by others—maybe your family members, past partners, work associates, or friends.

Tune into your back and become aware of how much baggage you are carrying. Allow yourself to release all the baggage, stress, or knives into a purple flame of light. You can do this by visualizing dense energy moving out of your back and into the purple flame, or by using your hands and physically taking the knives, stuckness, fear, and pain out of your body and throwing them into the flame.

Say: "Divine Healing Intelligence, I ask you to free my back from all the worry, anger, struggle, suffering, conflict, victimhood, and emotional and mental baggage I carry, as well as all points of view, all patterns, and the positive and negative charges that contribute to this condition." Repeat the word "CLEAR" until you feel a shift occur.

Imagine a beautiful gold light moving through your back, releasing any density and tension from it. When the tension has released, imagine yourself surrounded by green light, which will act as a support for your back and nervous system.

Say: "Divine Healing Intelligence, please install feelings and experiences of support, confidence, self-belief, trust, freedom, abundance, and success. Thank you."

Say: "Divine Healing Intelligence, please heal and regenerate my back and all related organs to their maximum strength, vitality, and flexibility. Thank you."

Unhealthy emotions to work with (page 171): Worry 197, Anger 173, Stress 194, Frustration 181, Feeling Overwhelmed 180
Healthy emotions to work with (page 197): Peace 204, Support 206, Success 207
Colors to work with (page 211): Gold 213, Green 213

## *Bladder*

### Possible Contributing Factors

Feeling timid, wishy-washy, inefficient, annoyed, irritable, sad, and guilty. Sense of powerlessness and frustration. Feeling angry or "pissed off" with a partner or person you are close to. Wanting to be somewhere else other than where you are. Holding on to worries from the past, which stop you from moving forward. Lack of boundaries. Needing your own space.

### Remedy

Inhale deeply several times. Place your hands on your bladder and tune into what you are feeling. Are you angry, pissed off, or irritated with someone or something in your life? Are you allowing this irritation to control your life?

Say: "Divine Healing Intelligence, I ask you to dissolve all feelings of anger, indecisiveness, weakness, irritability, powerlessness, and worry from my bladder, as well as all points of view, all patterns, and the positive and negative charges that contribute to this condition." Repeat the word "CLEAR" until you feel a shift occur.

Rub your hands together. Place the palms of your hands slightly apart, feeling the tingling sensation. Imagine that you hold in your hands a yellow ball of healing energy. Ask the Divine Healing Intelligence to make this ball of energy stronger. You may even see or sense rays of golden sunlight energizing this ball, making it more powerful and effective.

Place your hands on your bladder, allowing the ball to penetrate deeply into your bladder. Focus on the warmth emanating from this golden ball as it dissolves and purifies the physical, emotional, and mental density and tension in the bladder. Observe it until the bladder comes back into perfect health and vitality.

Say: "Divine Healing Intelligence, please install feelings and experiences of confidence, certainty, determination, harmony, happiness, humor, and joy. Thank you."

To make the process even more powerful, gently hum the vowel sound "OOO" (as in the word "you") and direct the sound toward the bladder. Allow the sound to infuse your bladder with healing and balancing energy. Hum for a minute or two.

Say: "Divine Healing Intelligence, please heal and regenerate my bladder and all related organs to their maximum strength, vitality, and well-being. Thank you."

Unhealthy emotions to work with (page 171): Anger 173, Resentment 192, Sadness 193, Frustration 181

Healthy emotions to work with (page 197): Forgiveness 200, Happiness 201, Confidence 198

Colors to work with (page 211): Yellow 221, Green 213

## *Blood*

### Possible Contributing Factors

Experiencing tension, unhappiness, rejection, guilt, shame, suspicion, and resistance. Difficulty communicating with a partner, family member, close friend, or coworker. Suppressing your creativity. Disregarding your dreams and desires. Carrying ancestral fears and your own stresses that can add to or exacerbate blood disorders. Suffering from a lack of self-esteem and feelings of incompetence. Loss of life's meaning through trauma or loss. In children, feeling conflicted or unsupported. Taking responsibility for the arguments and fights of the parents.

### Remedy

In order to regenerate and purify the blood, focus on bright red. Imagine that you are directing this bright red ray all through your body, starting from your toes and moving it through your feet, legs, thighs, torso, head, and back down again. Become aware of where the blood feels stuck and is not flowing freely. Intensify the color in that area. You may feel warmth or tingling. Allow the bright red ray to become a vacuum that sucks in and then dissolves all the density it finds. If the energy feels blocked in your arms, hands, legs, or feet, start shaking them gently to stir the blood and help it flow.

To eliminate problems with the blood, you can also vigorously massage that area of your body, or even take a hair brush and brush your skin until it becomes pink and tingly.

Say: "Divine Healing Intelligence, I ask you to dissolve all tension, unhappiness, resistance, rejection, fears, upsets, and stresses out of my blood, as well as all points of view, all patterns, and the positive and negative charges that contribute to this condition." Repeat the word "CLEAR" until you feel a shift occur.

Say: "Divine Healing Intelligence, please intensify my ability to communicate clearly and openly with others. Help me experience joy, laughter, happiness, and peace. Allow me to be free to express myself and allow my creativity to flourish. Thank you."

Focus on awakening the blood further by intensifying the heat with the red ray and then cooling it down with a blue ray. Do this eight to ten times. Move through the whole body, heating then cooling it.

Say: "Divine Healing Intelligence, please heal and regenerate my blood to its maximum strength, vitality, and purity. Thank you."

Unhealthy emotions to work with (page 171): Rejection 191, Guilt 184, Shame 193, Fear 179, Stress 194, Low Self-Esteem 190

Healthy emotions to work with (page 197): Forgiveness 200, Joy 203, Compassion 198, Confidence 198

Colors to work with (page 211): Red 218, Blue 211, Violet 220, Green 213, Indigo 214

## Bones

### Possible Contributing Factors

Self-imposed limitation, resentment, inflexibility, bitterness, and blame. Degeneration of bones due to not honoring yourself and your body. Hardening bones as a result of being hard on yourself and expecting too much of yourself and others. Weakening of bones related to feelings of being lost, disempowered, isolated, worried, stressed, ashamed, or unkind. Breaks occurring during breaking points in your life, from deep-seated pain, or when you feel the need to hurt or punish yourself.

## Remedy

Take a clear glass and wrap a sheet of orange cellophane around it. Pour some water into the glass. Place your hands over the water and say, "Divine Spirit, please infuse this water with binding, healing, and regenerative energy. Please energize the crystals in the water with mending and repairing qualities so that my bones may heal and become stronger and more resilient. Thank you."

Allow the glass of water to take in the orange light. Place it in the sunlight. After a few hours, drink it very slowly. With every sip, imagine that the orange liquid is cleansing and repairing your bones.

Say: "Divine Healing Intelligence, I ask you to release all self-imposed limitation, hardness, resentment, inflexibility, bitterness, and blame from my bones, as well as all points of view, all patterns, and the positive and negative charges that contribute to this condition." Repeat the word "CLEAR" until you feel a shift occur.

Say: "Divine Healing Intelligence, please install inner strength, confidence, self-belief, appreciation, and acceptance. Help me to be kind, loving, and to honor myself and others. Thank you."

Repeat this process every day for a month or for as long as it takes to improve the strength of your bones.

If you have a fractured bone, imagine that green light surrounds the bone, allowing it to mend.

Say: "Divine Healing Intelligence, please heal and regenerate my bones to their maximum strength, vitality, and flexibility. Thank you."

Unhealthy emotions to work with (page 171): Anger 173, Resentment 192, Sadness 193, Frustration 181

Healthy emotions to work with (page 197): Forgiveness 200, Flexibility and Movement 200, Peace 204, Satisfaction 206

Colors to work with (page 211): Orange 216, Green 213, Violet 220

## *Bowels*

### Possible Contributing Factors

Difficulty letting go of old, outdated beliefs. Judging others as wrong and yourself as right. An "It's my way or the highway" attitude. Desire to control others, thinking, *If only they would change, my life would be better.* Constantly telling others what to do and how to live their lives. Perfectionism. Refusal to listen to other peoples' suggestions. Feeling stuck, frustrated, and fearful of change. Fear of the unknown.

### Remedy

For problems with constipation or diarrhea, slowly massage your index fingers on both hands, from the base to the tip, using the index finger and thumb of the opposite hand. Do this for a few minutes on each hand. Take slow, deep breaths as you massage.

Close your eyes and picture a yellow ray of light moving through your intestines, cleansing them of any waste and toxicity.

Ask yourself the following questions to help clarify what you are holding on to:

*Am I holding on to a relationship that has run its course?*
*Am I holding on to a job that I need to leave?*
*Am I holding on to pain from the past?*
*Am I holding on to anger from the past?*

Continue to ask yourself similar questions. When you recognize that you are clinging to a destructive pattern, habit, person, or situation, clench your fists and allow yourself to fully feel what it is like to hold on. Ask yourself, *Can anything else come into my life when I hold on to negativity?*

Say: "Divine Healing Intelligence, I ask you to release all judgment, criticism, righteous attitude, perfectionism, fear of change, and feeling of stuckness from my bowels, as well as all points of view, all patterns, and the positive and negative charges that contribute to this condition." Repeat the word "CLEAR" until you feel a shift occur.

Open your fists and allow your palms to relax. When you feel ready to let go, just blow the density and tension out of your hands. Feel what it is like to release stuckness and stagnation from your life. Ask yourself, *What amazing opportunities are available to me now?*

Say: "Divine Healing Intelligence, please intensify my ability to change my life for the better. Help me to welcome healing, uplifting and Divine experiences into my life. Thank you."

If you have further problems with constipation, try the following process: Find the indent in the middle of your chin using your fingertips on one hand (palm facing you). Place your middle finger on that spot while keeping your other fingers straight and your palm flat. Massage your chin in a small circular motion as firmly as possible for forty-five seconds. Rest and then repeat the process two or three times. Visualize your bowels surrounded with revitalizing green light.

Say: "Divine Healing Intelligence, please heal and regenerate my bowels and all related organs to their maximum strength, vitality, and well-being. Thank you."

Unhealthy emotions to work with (page 171): Stuckness 196, Judgment 188, Control 174, Fear 179

Healthy emotions to work with (page 197): Flexibility and Movement 200, Freedom 201, Relaxation 205

Colors to work with (page 211): Brown 212, Yellow 221, Green 213

## *Brain*

### Possible Contributing Factors

Neglecting your body's computer by downloading mental viruses in the form of negative thoughts, worries, and stresses. Feeling out of control, depressed, bored, flat, disinterested, disheartened, and sleepy. Feeling like your mind is hazy, scattered, conflicted, or confused.

## Remedy

Close your eyes. Focus on your brain. Consciously relax your head. Hum the sound "EEE" (as in the word "me") for one to two minutes. This sound helps the brain relax, and become clearer and more receptive. Do this helpful exercise before studying, taking a test, learning a new skill, or making an important decision.

Imagine that the brain is a computer with various programs running at once. Focus on belief systems or programs that no longer serve you. Then imagine a computer screen in your brain with this particular program or belief written on the screen. Picture a "delete" key and press it. Allow yourself to completely erase the negative program from the screen.

Say: "Divine Healing Intelligence, I ask you to dissolve from my brain all negative thoughts and programs; all worries, stresses, depression, boredom, and haziness; as well as all points of view, all patterns, and the positive and negative charges that contribute to this condition." Repeat the word "CLEAR" until you feel a shift occur.

If you would like to write some new programs to replace the ones you deleted, imagine yourself typing new, positive beliefs onto the computer screen and saving them.

Say: "Divine Healing Intelligence, please install clarity, trust, peace, creativity, and self-expression. Allow me to make the most empowered decisions quickly, easily, and effortlessly. Thank you."

Take some very deep breaths and imagine the color purple surrounding your brain. Allow this color to release any residue of stagnation and bring you clarity, courage, and success.

In order to improve your concentration and memory, and to sharpen your mind, try the following: Touch the tip of your thumb to the tip of your index finger and stretch out the other fingers. Do this to both hands for two to five minutes, several times a day.

Say: "Divine Healing Intelligence, please heal and regenerate my brain and all related organs to their maximum health, vitality, and well-being. Thank you."

Unhealthy emotions to work with (page 171): Criticism 175, Judgment 188, Control 174, Stuckness 196
Healthy emotions to work with (page 197): Clarity 197, Relaxation 205, Freedom 201
Colors to work with (page 211): Purple 217, Violet 220, Yellow 221

## Breasts

### Possible Contributing Factors
A lack of nurturing, gentle love for yourself while showering it onto others. Believing that you don't deserve to receive from others or to be supported.

### Right Breast
Never still, always busy doing things. Propensity to become a workaholic. Difficulty saying no. Thinking that if you don't do something, the world might end. Trying to please everyone and then feeling torn in different directions. Sometimes carrying the archetype of a slave. Often feeling like a victim. Asking yourself, *Why does this happen to me?* Holding on to childhood hurts from your family. Feeling overwhelmed and overpowered by others. Trying to be too controlling in order not to fall apart. Easily trapped in an abusive relationship. Often carrying anger toward men and the pain they have caused. Sadness about a failed relationship. For parents, disappointment and hurt that you don't have the relationship you desire with your kids.

### Left Breast
Difficulty connecting to your own femininity and receiving love, affection, and kindness. Feeling like you don't need help from others because you can take care of everything yourself. Overburdening yourself with responsibilities and then pushing yourself beyond your limits, feeling anxious and exhausted. Not having any clear boundaries. Holding on to rejection, shame, disappointment, insecurity, and fear. Always worrying about everyone and everything. Deep need to be liked and to please others. Deep fear of loss. Regret about the choices you have made. Living in the past and wishing that things were different.

## Remedy

Focus on your breasts. Do you love, appreciate, and look after them? Or do you criticize them; poke fun at them; or carry disappointment, hurt, and shame in your breasts and chest? Stand in front of the mirror, take off your top, and look at your breasts. Focus on letting go of all criticism, and see them from a new perspective of love and appreciation.

With your hands, take out any density, energetic knives, ropes, or abuse from your breasts and put them into an imaginary fire. Allow them to release on all levels until your breasts feel nice and light inside.

Say: "Divine Healing Intelligence, I ask you to help me release hardness, disappointment, disconnection from my own needs, feelings of rejection, tiredness, loss, and victimhood from my breasts, as well as all points of view, all patterns, and the positive and negative charges that contribute to this condition." Repeat the word "CLEAR" until you feel a shift occur.

Cup your breasts in the palms of your hands and focus on sending green, healing, rejuvenating light into your breasts. Then hug yourself, focusing on loving and nurturing your breasts.

Complete the following sentence: "I love my breasts because _____." Repeat this five times, telling your breasts all the different reasons you love them. It could be anything:

*My breasts give me pleasure.*
*They make me feel more feminine.*
*I was or am able to nurture my children with my breasts.*

Say: "Divine Healing Intelligence, please help me love, nurture, and listen to myself. Help me to have a balanced outlook on life, increase my inner power, and allow me the freedom to be myself. Thank you."

Do something loving and nurturing every day, even if it only takes a moment. Smile at yourself, give yourself a compliment, rest, read, dance, or do whatever feels right.

Say: "Divine Healing Intelligence, please heal and regenerate my breasts and all related organs to their maximum health, vitality, and well-being. Thank you."

## *Buttocks*

### Possible Contributing Factors

Feelings of distrust, disappointment, lack of self-esteem and possibilities, fear, ignorance, and loss of power. Lack of stability and security. Holding on to stress, old stubborn anger, and guilt. Loss of sexual energy or feeling unattractive. Feeling stuck and fearful of new experiences, your own wisdom, and your innate ability to create.

### Remedy

Many people walk all day with very tight buttocks, holding on to stress, fear, and tension. Consciously focus on relaxing your buttocks. You can do this by slowly breathing in and tightening your buttocks while you hold your breath for five seconds. Then relax your buttocks as you slowly breathe out. Repeat this process eight to ten times. Then gently massage the buttocks or shake them out until they feel more relaxed. Check regularly to see if they are tight or relaxed, and do this exercise any time there is tension.

Say: "Divine Healing Intelligence, I ask you to melt all resentment, sexual tension, distrust, disappointment, lack, fear, ignorance, anger, guilt, and loss of power out of my buttocks as well as all points of view, all patterns, and the positive and negative charges that contribute to this condition." Repeat the word "CLEAR" until you feel a shift occur.

Every day for a week, look at your behind in the mirror and compliment it. Find all the things you like about it. Say to yourself, "I love my bottom" or "I love my buttocks." Saying this will allow your lower back and hips to relax more, relieve tension, and ease any pain and difficulty in walking.

Say: "Divine Healing Intelligence, please install a sense of stability, innocence, and enjoyment of my sensuality. Allow me to experience fun, playfulness, and pleasure. Thank you."

Say: "Divine Healing Intelligence, please heal and regenerate my buttocks and all related organs to their maximum health, vitality, and well-being. Thank you."

Unhealthy emotions to work with (page 171): Fear 179, Stress 194, Anger 173, Guilt 184

Healthy emotions to work with (page 197): Forgiveness 200, Innocence 202, Relaxation 205, Joy 203

Colors to work with (page 211): Orange 216, Green 213, Blue 211, Red 218

## Cervix

### Possible Contributing Factors

Out of flow with life. Disconnected from your feminine energy. Feeling victimized, overpowered, attacked, manipulated, abused, taken for granted. Conflict in close relationships. Difficulty letting go of old ways of being and giving birth to new experiences. Lacking affection, love, and nurturing. Grief about dreams that have not manifested. Being told that you can't do something that is important to you. Feeling imprisoned.

### Remedy

To heal, you need to allow yourself to reconnect with the flow of life. Ask yourself, *Where am I out of flow with who I am? How am I not listening to my own guidance and allowing others to run my life?*

Become aware of where in your life you are harsh, critical, and hard on yourself. Take slow, deep breaths and visualize blazing orange sunlight. Imagine melting any hardness, criticism, and resistance you have in your reproductive system, heart, and other parts of your body.

Say: "Divine Healing Intelligence, I ask you to melt away all resistance, victimhood, manipulation, fear, ignorance, conflict, and abuse from my cervix as well as all

31

points of view, all patterns, and the positive and negative charges that contribute to this condition." Repeat the word "CLEAR" until you feel a shift occur.

Rub your hands together. Place them slightly apart. Visualize a beautiful pink light coming out of your hands. Place your hands on your lower abdomen. Take a slow, deep breath in. Feel this soft, sweet pink light move into your body and soften it. If you feel comfortable, hum the sound "VAM" (VAAAAAAAAAHHHHHHHMM MMMMM) for a few minutes.

Say: "Divine Healing Intelligence, please install a sense of softness, support, and enjoyment of my sensuality and pleasure. Allow me to come back into alignment with myself and listen to my own wisdom. Thank you."

Sit up straight. Clasp your hands with your fingers intertwined. Place your left thumb on top of the right. Place your hands at the level of your lower abdomen. Hold this position for five minutes while breathing in qualities of confidence, joy, creativity, and self-love. Allow yourself to relax as much as possible.

Say: "Divine Healing Intelligence, please heal and regenerate my cervix and all related organs to their maximum health, vitality, and well-being. Thank you."

Unhealthy emotions to work with (page 171): Fear 179, Grief 182, Resentment 192, Criticism 175

Healthy emotions to work with (page 197): Compassion 198, Forgiveness 200, Love 203, Joy 203

Colors to work with (page 211): Orange 216, Pink 217, Yellow 221

## Chest

### Possible Contributing Factors

Experiencing heaviness, as if you are carrying a burden or weight on your chest. Giving too much of your energy and self to others without much reciprocation. Feeling disempowered, tired, empty, fearful, anxious, and worn out. Difficulty expressing your feelings. Trying to control people and situations to feel safe and then feeling stifled and restricted. Lack of self-trust, spontaneity, and creativity.

## Remedy

Sit or lie down. Breathe slowly and deeply, allowing your body to completely relax. Imagine lying in a bath of healing orange liquid. Allow your body to soften and enjoy the experience. Sense or imagine a funnel in the middle of your chest.

Say: "Divine Healing Intelligence, I ask you to release all burdens, disempowerment, low self-esteem, suppression of feelings, anxiety, and fear from my chest, as well as all points of view, all patterns, and the positive and negative charges that contribute to this condition." Repeat the word "CLEAR" until you feel a shift occur.

Say: "I allow all the cells in my body that are experiencing heaviness, degeneration, infection, or stress to now be released through this funnel into a purple flame."

Observe as toxic and heavy energy moves out of your body, through the funnel, and into the purple flame. Using your thumb, gently massage the point between your ring finger and middle finger, on the palm of your right hand. Massage it gently in a slow circular motion for a minute or two. While you are massaging, take deep, slow breaths, allowing your chest to fill with oxygen, and then expel all impurities from your chest and lungs. Do the same while massaging in the same place and fashion on your left hand.

Say: "Divine Healing Intelligence, please install a way for me to experience a life of ease, freedom, creativity, and love. Help me to find peace and tranquility in my heart and soul. Thank you."

Say: "Divine Healing Intelligence, please heal and regenerate my chest, lungs, and heart to their maximum strength, vitality, and well-being. Thank you."

Unhealthy emotions to work with (page 171): Anxiety 174, Control 174, Low Self-Esteem 190
Healthy emotions to work with (page 197): Peace 204, Relaxation 205, Confidence 198, Freedom 201
Colors to work with (page 211): Orange 216, Turquoise 219, Gold 213

## *Ears*

### Possible Contributing Factors

Blocking what you don't want to hear. Not listening to your own guidance and wisdom. Holding on to anger, frustration, blame, guilt, resentment. Mishearing or misunderstanding people. Refusal to change your mind or broaden your perspective. Feeling out of balance, dizzy, unaware, unnerved.

### *Right Ear*

Feeling impatient, angry, annoyed, hurt by other people's comments. Involved in too much conflict or too many arguments. Feel like you've had an earful. Holding on to destructive beliefs from the past, especially childhood, and replaying them. Feeling tired, worn out; dispirited about your life, work, family, and environment.

### *Left Ear*

Feeling that what you have to say is not important, and not worth hearing or listening to. Spending time around people who judge and criticize you. Criticizing yourself.

### Remedy

Your ears are like sponges that absorb information. There are so many sounds you are unaware of because you are only able to focus on small amounts of information at a time. Much of what we hear is negative. This negativity has the ability to affect not only your ears but many other parts of your body. Start becoming aware of the noise around you and how it is affecting your ears. Does it make you want to block your ears and run away, or does it make you want to sit up and listen?

Ask yourself, *Is there anything I don't want to hear?* Next time you are around someone who is saying something hurtful or upsetting, imagine indigo rays moving through your left ear to push anything that is dense or unclear out through your right ear and into a fire that dissipates the negativity. Repeat the process for the other ear.

Say: "Divine Healing Intelligence, I ask you to dissolve all negativity, guilt, anger, resentment, stuckness, frustration, and criticism out of my ears, as well as all points of view, all patterns, and the positive and negative charges that contribute to this condition." Repeat the word "CLEAR" until you feel a shift occur.

Lightly massage the little finger on your right hand from the root to the tip using small circular movements. Then do the same with the little finger on your left hand.

The ear contains more than a hundred acupoints, which can stimulate life force energy and reinvigorate your body. Massage the lobes of both ears with your thumbs and index fingers. Start at the top of the lobes and massage slowly for about a minute.

Sit up. Hold your earlobes. Now pull them down for about a minute. Relax and breathe deeply for thirty seconds, then repeat this process three times. This will help to release tension, exhaustion, and stress from your body.

Put your hands gently over your ears. Ask to hear your own wisdom and guidance, then breathe slowly and listen. Practice this regularly to have perfect hearing and to listen to your own wisdom.

To improve your hearing, place your thumbs on top of your middle fingers, while keeping the other fingers straight. Hold this position for about five minutes. If you have an earache, do this several times a day.

Say: "Divine Healing Intelligence, please install a way for me to experience harmony, peace, clarity, balance, increased self-esteem, love, and appreciation. Thank you."

Say: "Divine Healing Intelligence, please heal and regenerate my ears and hearing abilities to their maximum capacity and well-being. Thank you."

Unhealthy emotions to work with (page 171): Guilt 184, Resentment 192, Anger 173, Shame 193, Criticism 175
Healthy emotions to work with (page 197): Forgiveness 200, Innocence 202, Joy 203, Respect 205, Satisfaction 206
Colors to work with (page 211): Mauve 215, Indigo 214, Violet 220

## *Elbows*

### Possible Contributing Factors

Stagnation, limitation, frustration, anger, jealousy. Lacking awareness of your own needs. Stiffness in mind and body, the belief that life is all struggle and strain. Lack of direction.

### *Right Elbow*

Feeling elbowed, poked, and jabbed by others. People interfering in your life. Feeling tormented, harassed, taken advantage of, made fun of, taken for a ride. Difficulty letting go of old hurts and anger.

### *Left Elbow*

Feeling unsupported and weak. Leaning too much on others. Difficulty making decisions. Feeling stressed and overwhelmed. Either overemotional or suppressing feelings.

### Remedy

Say: "Divine Healing Intelligence, I ask you to dissolve all stagnation, stiffness, struggle, strain, weakness, tension, hurt, and anger from my elbows, as well as all points of view, all patterns, and the positive and negative charges that contribute to this condition." Repeat the word "CLEAR" until you feel a shift occur.

Rub your hands together for forty-five seconds. Place your hands apart. Visualize a green ball of energy in the palms of your hands. Place your hand on the affected elbow. Hold it there while visualizing green light entering and regenerating your elbow. Repeat "Heal, mend, regenerate now" for two to three minutes until you feel lighter.

Say: "Divine Healing Intelligence, please install awareness, self-belief, a clear direction for me to follow, feelings of support, inner strength, and freedom. Thank you."

Say: "Divine Healing Intelligence, please heal and regenerate my elbows, arms, hands, and bones to their maximum strength, flexibility, and well-being. Thank you."

*See also* Arms.

Unhealthy emotions to work with (page 171): Frustration 181, Anger 173, Jealousy 187

Healthy emotions to work with (page 197): Flexibility and Movement 200, Faith 199, Recognition 204, Confidence 198

Colors to work with (page 211): Green 213, Yellow 221, Silver 219

## Eyes

### Possible Contributing Factors

Not liking what you are seeing in your environment. Suspicious of people and events. Seeing obstacles and limitations. Wanting things to be different. Fixation on aging. Seeing life from a negative point of view. Feeling stuck. Seeing things from only one direction or perspective. Fearful of the future. Wanting what others have.

### *Right Eye*

Blocking the flow of abundance and prosperity. Experiencing challenges in your relationships. Not seeing how you can change this situation. Holding on to pain from the past and projecting it onto the future. Making excuses and finding reasons why things won't work. Irritated with yourself and others.

### *Left Eye*

Difficulty visualizing good things in your life. Seeing only the negative or challenging parts of your existence. Experiencing a lack of joy, fun, and creativity. Believing that life is chaotic, hard, challenging, and full of struggles and seeking proof of this. Focusing on pain, lack, and limitation. Losing trust that life will provide for you by upholding fear, stress, and worry.

### Remedy

Are there things you are seeing that you don't want to see? For example, are you seeing someone close to you suffering or unhappy? Do you keep trying to make them happy, and then feel hopeless and defeated because they won't change? If you desire your vision to improve, you need to shift your focus from what you don't want to see to what makes you feel happy and brings beauty into your life. You can go for nature walks, spend time by the ocean, visit people who inspire you, or be creative by painting beautiful pictures in your mind and on paper.

Go outside into the light. Close your eyes. Place the palms of your hands over your eyes. Allow the healing energy of sunlight to work on regenerating your eyes. Do this for a few minutes, two to three times a day.

Relax your hands. Open your eyes and look at the sky's beautiful rays of blue light. Even if the sky is gray, find where it has glimmers of blue light. Close your eyes and visualize blue rays of light moving through your eyes, washing all density, degeneration, stuckness, or hardness from them. Allow your eyes to relax and soften even further before opening them.

Open your eyes. Spend thirty seconds blinking frequently to allow moisture to return.

In order to improve your vision, you also need to improve the eyes' flexibility. Rotate the eyes to the left, to the right, and then up and down. Do this eight to ten times. Repeat the process, rotating your eyes to the right, to the left, down, and then up. Do this also eight to ten times. If you suffer from cataracts, try wearing transparent indigo-colored glasses so that the light can enter and regenerate your eyes.

Say: "Divine Healing Intelligence, I ask you to release all anger, suspicion, distrust, and frustration from my past. Assist me in dissolving all the stress, irritation, negativity, hardness, fear, obstacles, and projected problems from my eyes, as well as all points of view, all patterns, and the positive and negative charges that contribute to this condition." Repeat the word "CLEAR" until you feel a shift occur.

Say: "Divine Healing Intelligence, please install feelings and experiences of clarity, trust, patience, relaxation, softness, flexibility, and peace. Thank you."

Say: "Divine Healing Intelligence, please heal and regenerate my eyes and all related organs to their maximum strength, vitality, and flexibility. Thank you."

Unhealthy emotions to work with (page 171): Fear 179, Stress 194, Worry 197, Jealousy 187, Frustration 181

Healthy emotions to work with (page 197): Clarity 197, Compassion 198, Peace 204, Forgiveness 200

Colors to work with (page 211): Purple 217, Blue 211, Indigo 214, Violet 220, Mauve 215

## *Face*

### Possible Contributing Factors

Repeating the same old destructive patterns, stressing, frowning, limiting yourself, struggling, and feeling disconnected from your heart and soul. Fear of rejection. Not taking the opportunity to truly know yourself, limiting your ability to face challenging situations successfully. Losing face.

### Remedy

Look at your face in the mirror. Spend five minutes seeing all the things you like and appreciate about your face.

Now look more deeply at what your face is trying to tell you. Are you facing situations courageously or hiding behind a mask? Does your face tell a happy story or a story of struggle, fear, and strain?

Decide to face situations which need attention head on, instead of hiding from them or pretending they don't exist. This may mean confronting someone you've been avoiding, paying off your debts, or finally starting a project you have been procrastinating with. Whatever it is, start taking steps toward resolving conflicting and stagnant situations.

Spend a few minutes massaging your face gently and lovingly. You may use a natural cream or oil to rub into your skin. Then close your eyes and imagine you have a trash bin in front of you. Picture yourself taking off any false masks that are covering your face, and throw them in the bin until you get to the most beautiful, shining face that you would like to show the world. Repeat this exercise twice a day for a few weeks.

Say: "Divine Healing Intelligence, I direct you to release all strain, stress, false masks, old fashioned beliefs, and struggles from my face, as well all points of view, all patterns, and the positive and negative charges that contribute to this condition." Repeat the word "CLEAR" until you feel a shift occur.

Say: "Divine Healing Intelligence, please bring to the surface my ability to face life with courage, faith, and inner strength. Allow me to lighten up, connect with my spirit, and find new, constructive ways to live my life. Bring to the surface my innocence, purity, and shining potential. Thank you."

If you would like to improve your complexion or if you have facial paralysis, work with this process daily. Bend your index finger. Place your thumb on top of your index finger. Extend the other fingers. Take slow, deep breaths. Hold the gesture for five minutes. If you have facial paralysis you may need to hold it for forty-five minutes.

Say: "Divine Healing Intelligence, please heal and regenerate my face and all related organs to their maximum health, vitality, and beauty. Thank you."

Unhealthy emotions to work with (page 171): Fear 179, Rejection 191, Failure 178, Stress 194, Stuckness 196
Healthy emotions to work with (page 197): Relaxation 205, Satisfaction 206, Confidence 198, Success 207, Joy 203
Colors to work with (page 211): Blue 211, Indigo 214, Purple 217, Pink 217

## Fallopian Tubes

### Possible Contributing Factors
Difficulty moving from one place to another. Feeling sadness, loss, shame, grief, depression. Carrying guilt or fear about children or childbirth. Afraid of losing your femininity or of becoming too old to have children.

### Remedy
Focus on your fallopian tubes. If you could see them, would they look clear and healthy or blocked and unhealthy? Ask yourself the following questions:

*What am I trying to suppress or stop from happening?"*
*How do I feel about my femininity?*

*How am I buying into other peoples' negative beliefs about aging and about my ability to create a healthy family?*

*Where am I stuck in my life?*

*What decisions, actions, and steps do I need to take to move forward?*

By asking the right questions, you can allow yourself to free up stuck or stagnant energy.

Focus on an orange ray of light. Visualize it moving through your fallopian tubes, dissolving all blockages and releasing degeneration. Focus on a yellow ray of light moving through your fallopian tubes, clearing and regenerating them to full health and vitality.

If you would like to have children, give yourself permission to be more fertile, creative, and feminine.

If you want children but are unable to have them, forgive your body for not being able to support you in that experience. Connect to your reproductive system and surround it with pink rays of love. Ask Divine Intelligence to bring children into your life through other means.

Say: "Divine Healing Intelligence, I ask you to release all stuckness, loneliness, shame, grief, depression, and feelings of loss from my fallopian tubes, as well as all points of view, all patterns, and the positive and negative charges that contribute to this condition." Repeat the word "CLEAR" until you feel a shift occur.

Say: "Divine Healing Intelligence, please help me to move ahead in life effortlessly; express my feminine nature fully; connect to my creativity; and bring back my sense of youth, vibrancy, and vitality. Thank you."

Say: "Divine Healing Intelligence, please heal and regenerate my fallopian tubes and all related organs to their maximum strength, vitality, and health. Thank you."

Unhealthy emotions to work with (page 171): Sadness 193, Shame 193, Depression 176, Resentment 192, Stuckness 196

Healthy emotions to work with (page 197): Forgiveness 200, Honor 202, Peace 204, Compassion 198

Colors to work with (page 211): Orange 216, Purple 217, Silver 219, Yellow 221

## *Feet*

### Possible Contributing Factors

Moving in the wrong direction; ignoring your intuition; feeling confused, lost, ungrounded, or out of touch with reality. Feeling stuck, bogged down, obligated to others; missing the big picture. Indecisiveness. Getting cold feet about a situation.

### *Right Foot*

Too much obligation; feeling angry, irritated, frustrated, and enraged. Focusing a great deal on material things and what you are going to get out of a situation. Trying to break through something using force rather than standing back and allowing it to happen. Shooting yourself in the foot.

### *Left Foot*

Disconnected from your needs. Too much focus on the outside world and what you need to do for others. Blockages in your path that lead to things not turning out the way you had intended. Dragging pain from the past or from difficult relationships. An imbalance between giving and receiving.

### Remedy

You have an opportunity to look at your life and change direction. Focus on letting go of things from the past and moving forward. Nurture yourself and appreciate your feet, which work very hard to carry you.

Take your left foot into your hands and massage it as if it were your most precious and valuable asset. Would you sell your foot for a million dollars? Most likely not. Begin to value it and treat it as the extremely important part of your life that it is. Then change over and massage your right foot.

Feet carry us around every day. They hold us up and support our weight. Feet also have a connection to the Earth and an ability to release a lot of dense energy.

Stand and imagine that your feet have two big ducts through which all dense energy can release and dissolve into the Earth, where it can be transmuted. Now, focus on what you would like to release from your feet. Move your feet and shake the tension, fear, limitation, and stress out through them.

Say: "Divine Healing Intelligence, I ask you to release all stuckness, limitation, burdens, anger, irritation, frustration, and neglect from my feet, as well as all points of view, all patterns, and the positive and negative charges that contribute to this condition." Repeat the word "CLEAR" until you feel a shift occur.

Stand. Focus on moving toward your dreams. Imagine that there are actual steps you can take toward your success. Give yourself permission to be successful. Now, take the steps forward. Each time you take a step, stop and breathe. Become aware of how much easier it is to succeed at that step than the previous one. Feel success, which can relate to well-being, work, family, love, money, and so forth. Then move forward.

Say: "Divine Healing Intelligence, please help me to move forward with ease and grace, and to be guided by Divine Wisdom. Allow me to be grounded, happy, clear, and more balanced. Thank you."

Say: "Divine Healing Intelligence, please heal and regenerate my feet, legs, and toes to their maximum health and mobility."

Unhealthy emotions to work with (page 171): Anger 173, Irritation 187, Frustration 181, Control 174, Stuckness 196

Healthy emotions to work with (page 197): Flexibility and Movement 200, Clarity 197, Support 206, Freedom 201

Colors to work with (page 211): Pink 217, Green 213, Brown 212

## *Fingers*

### Possible Contributing Factors

Inability to touch, hold, let go, give, and receive. Problems connecting to five of the major chakras in the body: root, sacral, solar plexus, heart, and throat.

*Right Hand*

**Thumb**—Connects to the pineal and pituitary glands in the brain, with the ability to restore equilibrium. Problems with a lack of creative power, sexual energy, and drive in life. Feeling lost, uninspired, and listless. Lacking vitality and willpower. Problems with circulation and blood. Carrying stress and worry.

**Index finger**—Holds intellect and how you think about yourself, your life, and the world around you; the source in the quest for power. Problems with feeling controlling or being controlled. Experiencing a sense of fear, rejection, and dread. On a physical level, stomach pains or heartburn from difficulty digesting life.

**Middle finger**—Connects with personal power and the ability to deal with many of life's challenges; holds the key to learning how to take personal responsibility. Problems with weight gain that masks emotional pain, sadness, anger, fear, and resentment. Feeling out of control, exhausted, drained, and confused.

**Ring finger**—Contains many beliefs about relationships and vows, especially those with a partner and with others in close relationships; holds connection to others. Problems giving and receiving love. Complications with the thymus, thyroid, and adrenals.

**Little finger**—Stores sense of survival and security, where beliefs about family and tribe reside; warehouse for childhood lessons. Problems trusting yourself and others. Feelings of not being good enough, strong enough, or courageous enough.

*Left Hand*

**Thumb**—Connected to the throat chakra, gives the ability to be a powerful communicator. Problems with self-assertion and self-worth. Unwillingness to stand up for yourself. Suppressing your feelings. Breathing difficulties, sinusitis, colds and sore throats, feelings of loneliness, and emotional coldness and detachment.

**Index finger**—Linked with the heart chakra, holds sense of individuality, belonging, and vision of yourself; the source for connecting to intuition and inspiration. Complications with the large intestine, including abdominal pain, diarrhea, and constipation.

**Middle finger**—Connected to the solar plexus chakra, maintains a sense of expansion, and the ability to take action and achieve results. Problems with painful experiences, judgments, criticisms, and perceived limitations of self. On a physical level, circulation and sexual problems.

**Ring finger**—Connected to the sacral chakra, holds connection to your inner child. Experiencing guilt, blame, shame, or anger, as well as feeling out of balance, stressed, unstable, or run-down. Problems with addictions lower back pain, fertility problems, and unresolved pain from childhood.

**Little finger**—Connected to the root chakra, affects self-esteem, how you fit into the world, and your rights. Problems connecting to your base or the Earth. Feeling unsafe or uncomfortable in own skin. Inability to create and achieve. Struggling with addictions, depression, lower back pain, or skin problems.

## Remedy

To release negative or dense energies and emotions from each finger, close your eyes and imagine that there is a fire in front of you. Using the fingers of the other hand, gently pull any dense issues out of the finger you are focusing on, and place the negativity (which may look like gray smoke, chains, or weeds) into the flame. You may then use the colors related to that specific finger to help regenerate the flow of energy:

- Thumb (throat chakra)—blue

- Index finger (heart chakra)—green

- Middle finger (solar plexus chakra)—yellow

- Ring finger (sacral chakra)—orange

- Little finger (root chakra)—red

In order to install and make the healthy emotions stronger, gently massage or hold each finger with the intention of increasing that feeling. Then bathe the finger in the color that relates to it. Do this slowly. If you are massaging, move from the base to tip, allowing yourself to really feel the positive emotion you are installing.

Say: "Divine Healing Intelligence, please heal and regenerate my fingers to their maximum health, vitality, and mobility."

Unhealthy emotions to work with (page 171): Any emotion that relates to the finger you are working on

Healthy emotions to work with (page 197): Any positive emotion that relates to the finger you are working on

Colors to work with (page 211): Colors related to the chakras or the color that you feel is most appropriate at the time

## Gallbladder

### Possible Contributing Factors

Resentment, grief about men, our masculine self, or achievement in the world. Feeling irritated, depressed, indecisive, confused, angry, wounded. Thinking of yourself as a failure, thus sabotaging opportunity for success. Feeling second best, neglected, unimportant, a victim. Holding on to trauma and pain from the past that creates struggles, hardship, and lack.

### Remedy

Focus on your gallbladder. What color do you imagine it to be? Is the color healthy or unhealthy?

The gallbladder is like a little bag that processes toxicity and density from the body. In your mind's eye, check if this bag is full or empty.

If it is full, concentrate on emptying the bag. Imagine throwing all the toxicity or stones into a purple fire. If you have gallstones, visualize dissolving them using red and orange rays of light. The red dissolves; the orange cleans up any residue.

Say: "Divine Healing Intelligence, I ask you to release all resentment, grief, self-sabotage, confusion, neglect, anger, and hurt from my gallbladder, as well as all points of view, all patterns, and the positive and negative charges that contribute to this condition." Repeat the word "CLEAR" until you feel a shift occur.

In your mind's eye, surround the gallbladder with green light. Allow the green light to move through the gallbladder and regenerate it. Place your hands on your gallbladder and focus on breathing slowly and deeply, allowing it to relax as much as possible.

Then, still holding your hands on your gallbladder, gently rub this area in a circular fashion. Repeat: "Heal, clear, and regenerate now," for about three minutes.

Say: "Divine Healing Intelligence, please intensify my ability to make clear, powerful, successful decisions. Allow my mind to open to experiencing abundance, ease, flow, and self-love. Thank you."

Say: "Divine Healing Intelligence, please heal and regenerate my gallbladder and all related organs to their maximum health, vitality, and well-being."

For the next few days, drink a lot of pure water and eat nutritious food to allow your gallbladder to detoxify and regenerate.

Unhealthy emotions to work with (page 171): Sadness 193, Stuckness 196, Resentment 192, Depression 176
Healthy emotions to work with (page 197): Compassion 198, Forgiveness 200, Honor 202, Faith 199, Success 207
Colors to work with (page 211): Orange 216, Red 218, Green 213

## Gums

### Possible Contributing Factors
Unsure of yourself and the decisions you have made. Not following through with projects, giving up too quickly, procrastinating. Too demanding and selfish. Refusing to change. Stuck, fearful, impatient, insecure, doubtful.

### Remedy
Close your eyes. Focus on your gums. Visualize a red ray of light moving through your gums, clearing and dissolving all infection, stagnation, and blockages. You might even feel your gums begin to tingle.

Say: "Divine Healing Intelligence, I ask you to release all procrastination, indecision, self-sabotage, selfishness, and stagnation from my gums, as well as all points of view, all patterns, and the positive and negative charges that contribute to this condition." Repeat the word "CLEAR" until you feel a shift occur.

Visualize a white ray of light moving through your gums, cleansing and regenerating them.

Massage your face and gums. Place the tips of your fingers above your mouth where you can feel your gums. Massage them for about sixty seconds. (If you find it difficult to massage with your fingers, do so with your knuckles.) Do this vigorously without hurting yourself. Rest for thirty seconds. If you are comfortable, massage for a further forty-five to sixty seconds. Then place the tips of your fingers below your lower lip where you can feel the gums. Repeat the procedure.

Say: "Divine Healing Intelligence, please guide me in making empowering decisions, following through with projects, being persistent, and opening myself to positive change and transformation. Thank you."

Say: "Divine Healing Intelligence, please heal and regenerate my gums and teeth to their maximum strength, vitality, and health."

Unhealthy emotions to work with (page 171): Irritation 187, Frustration 181, Fear 179, Stuckness 196

Healthy emotions to work with (page 197): Clarity 197, Confidence 198, Peace 204, Joy 203

Colors to work with (page 211): Red 218, White 220, Blue 211

## Hair

### Possible Contributing Factors

Issues with your insulation and protection. Trouble connecting to your beauty, creativity, self-worth, and self-love. Too much tension in the scalp from thinking; worrying; being afraid; and holding on to anger, frustration, guilt, resentment, or sadness, which results in hair loss or color change on a physical level—the body's way of showing you that what you are doing is not working.

### Remedy

Start by gently massaging your scalp using circular movements. As you do, imagine that rays of different colored lights are coming out of each of your fingers and that these rainbow-colored rays are stimulating the growth of your hair. As you massage, hold the intention of making your hair stronger, healthier, and more vibrant. Then imagine beautiful golden sunlight moving through your entire head of hair, making it smoother, softer, and shinier.

Say: "Divine Healing Intelligence, I ask you to delete all the stressful thoughts, worries, fears, anger, frustration, guilt, resentment, and sadness that are making my hair weak, as well as all points of view, all patterns, and the positive and negative charges that contribute to this condition." Repeat the word "CLEAR" until you feel a shift occur.

Lightly pull a tuft of your hair at the root to stimulate hair growth. Do this all over your head using both of your hands.

Say: "Divine Healing Intelligence, please help me gain self-belief, courage, and calmness, and increase my ability to trust that life has my best interests at hand. Allow me to recognize my own beauty and magnificence, and enjoy the gifts I have been given. Thank you."

Say: "Divine Healing Intelligence, please strengthen and regenerate my hair and scalp to their maximum health, vibrancy, and well-being."

Unhealthy emotions to work with (page 171): Stress 194, Fear 179, Criticism 175, Guilt 184

Healthy emotions to work with (page 197): Relaxation 205, Peace 204, Honor 202, Confidence 198

Colors to work with (page 211): White 220, Purple 217, Green 213, Magenta 215

## Hands

### Possible Contributing Factors

Inability to handle life. Repeatedly saying "I can't deal with things." Lending a helping hand to everybody else in need but yourself. Experiencing stiffness and fist clenching. Too much criticism and worry, which creates arthritic hands. Fear of the future, which creates hands that grip too tightly and lack faith in their ability to create. Healing hands gravitate toward healing others but cannot save the world; can only contribute to the lives of others if they are open to it.

### Right Hand

For many people, the dominant hand and the one with which they create. Problems with feeling lost, uncreative, fearful of the future. Experiencing struggle and frustration. Questions about ability to work, create money, and feed the family. Feeling disappointed or betrayed by someone considered a right-hand person or as someone's go-to person, helping and trusting only to be rejected.

### Left Hand

Holds more feminine energy. Complications from holding on to hurts from your family, mother, sister, wife, daughter, and so forth. Feeling isolated and lonely, not knowing how to take care of yourself, or how to find a clear path or direction. Resisting life and looking for handouts rather than taking charge, handling situations, and learning from these to become stronger and more empowered.

### Remedy

The palms of your hands have the ability to access Divine Healing Energy as well as healing energy from your body. Rub your hands together to activate your body's natural healing energy. Now, place them near each other and feel the tingling sensation.

Say: "I now activate my Divine Healing Energy."

Imagine that golden, healing light has been activated in the palms of your hands. Observe as this brilliant light expands and moves through your whole hand, clearing all blockages and toxicity from the blood and regenerating your hands.

Say: "Divine Healing Intelligence, I ask you to release all worry, inflexibility, control, resistance, loneliness, isolation, and tension I carry in my hands, as well as all points of view, all patterns, and the positive and negative charges that contribute to this condition." Repeat the word "CLEAR" until you feel a shift occur.

Shake or massage your hands for one to two minutes to help them to release any stuckness.

Link your fingers so that the palms of your hands are touching. Hold this hand position for a few moments, allowing the healing energy to grow and regenerate your hands.

Say: "Divine Healing Intelligence, please assist me to handle all situations with ease and grace, while taking responsibility for my actions. Help me learn from my life experiences and become more empowered. Thank you."

The more flexible and relaxed your hands are, the healthier your body will be. Hands contain many meridian points which relate to every organ in the body.

Say: "Divine Healing Intelligence, please heal and regenerate my hands, fingers, and wrists to their maximum health, strength, and flexibility."

Unhealthy emotions to work with (page 171): Control 174, Stuckness 196, Fear 179, Frustration 181

Healthy emotions to work with (page 197): Flexibility and Movement 200, Freedom 201, Confidence 198, Satisfaction 206

Colors to work with (page 211): Pink 217, Gold 213, Green 213

## *Head*

### Possible Contributing Factors

Feeling angry, frustrated, judgmental, self-critical, unaware, pigheaded. Stuck in a limited way of thinking and resistant to change. Overwhelmed by life, with too much to think about and too many burdens to carry. Always busy doing something or worrying about what you need to do. Perfectionism: "If it's going to be done right, it will be done my way." Loss of direction in life, forgetting what's important in life, and focusing on all your problems. Feeling like you need to control everyone and everything to be happy.

### Remedy

Focus on taking in deep breaths and relaxing your head. It may help you to relax more if you tighten your head, hold the tension for ten seconds, and then soften. Repeat this three to five times until your head feels lighter. Tilt back your head slightly, breathe in, and then slowly breathe out, bringing your head slightly forward. Do this for a few minutes.

Imagine that there is a lid on top of your head, which you can open to look inside. When you do, what do you see? Is it light or dark in there? Imagine that there is a light globe inside your head. If it is turned off, turn it on. Allow the light to move through your whole head as you focus on breathing deeply and relaxing even further.

Say: "Divine Healing Intelligence, I ask you to release all the overwhelming frustration, judgments, self-criticism, perfectionism, and stuckness from my head, as well as all points of view, all patterns, and the positive and negative charges that contribute to this condition." Repeat the word "CLEAR" until you feel a shift occur.

If you can, lie on a bed. Allow every muscle in your head and face to relax. Imagine that your head is completely weightless. Allow yourself to focus on yellow and white rays of light releasing the tension and stress from your head completely. Then gently hum the sound "EEE" (as in the word "me"), allowing the reverberation to clear your head even further. Now begin to focus on making decisions. You will find that your ideas and decisions become clearer, more creative, and more precise.

Say: "Divine Healing Intelligence, please allow me to be open to new ideas, experiences, and ways of thinking. Help me to become more flexible, aware, and clear about the choices I need to make."

Say: "Divine Healing Intelligence, please heal and regenerate my head and brain to their maximum health, vitality, and well-being."

Unhealthy emotions to work with (page 171): Judgment 188, Criticism 175, Feeling Overwhelmed 180, Worry 197

Healthy emotions to work with (page 197): Clarity 197, Peace 204, Relaxation 205, Happiness 201

Colors to work with (page 211): Indigo 214, Green 213, White 220, Yellow 221

## Heart

### Possible Contributing Factors

Feeling blocked, unenthusiastic, uninspired, flat, depressed, heavy-hearted, stressed. Thinking that life is too hard and you can't be bothered with dealing with it. Feeling closed-hearted, wounded, rejected, hardened, cold. Giving up on love, not believing you deserve it. Frequent self-criticism and self-deprecation. Feeling worthless, angry, and bitter. Waiting until things come to a boil to let your feelings out. Taking on too much responsibility, then feeling stressed and anxious. Giving too much of yourself and pushing yourself further than you can handle. Not listening to your heart. Feeling unfulfilled, disappointed, put-down, and lonely. Holding on to a deep-seated fear of being hurt or having your heart broken. In some cases, envy or jealousy over other people's success.

## Remedy

Close your eyes. Tune into your heart. Visualize your heart in your mind's eye. How does it look? Is it happy and expanded, joyfully giving and receiving love? Or is it constricted, stressed, tired, and limited?

Imagine that you have a hose in your hands that contains a clear healing liquid. Use this hose to wash away all grayness, density, and stress from your heart.

Say: "Divine Healing Intelligence, I ask you to delete all blockages, depression, heaviness, boredom, victimhood, anger, feelings of rejection, and stagnation from my heart, as well as all points of view, all patterns, and the positive and negative charges that contribute to this condition." Repeat the word "CLEAR" until you feel a shift occur.

Imagine the most beautiful rose-colored light, containing the energy of unconditional love, tenderness, and kindness. Allow the loving energy from this magnificent light to pour into your heart. Feel how your heart begins to soften, melting away any hardness or protection. Allow your heart's unconditional love to protect you. Even if your heart has experienced hurt, trust that it has developed wisdom and will now lead you to the most loving experiences possible.

Say: "Dear Heart, I want you to know how important you are to me. You work endlessly to keep me alive. You give me the opportunity to feel deeply; to experience love, joy, happiness; and to appreciate my life. I would like to say a deep, profound 'thank you' for the magnificent work that you do."

To intensify the love in your heart, rub your hands together and imagine the most beautiful magenta light coming out of them. Then relax your hands, and when you begin to feel a tingling sensation, place them on your heart to allow their warmth and the magenta light to envelop it.

Say: "Divine Healing Intelligence, please intensify my ability to listen to my heart's wisdom and follow its guidance. Allow my heart to open to love, kindness, affection, passion, fun, and deep joy. Thank you."

Say: "Divine Healing Intelligence, please heal and regenerate my heart and all related organs to their maximum health, vitality, and well-being."

Unhealthy emotions to work with (page 171): Depression 176, Stuckness 196, Judgment 188, Jealousy 187, Hatred 185, Fear 179

Healthy emotions to work with (page 197): Love 203, Happiness 201, Joy 203, Freedom 201, Peace 204

Colors to work with (page 211): Mauve 215, Magenta 215, Pink 217, Green 213

## Heels

### Possible Contributing Factors

Confusion, internal conflict, doubt. Questioning the essence of who you are. Second-guessing your decisions. A great need to stop and reevaluate your life. Out of flow and balance with life. Feeling like you have lost your strength and grounding. Walking on tiptoes around other people rather than saying what is really going on.

### Remedy

Massage your heels for a few minutes. Give yourself permission to stand your ground, take your place, and reclaim your confidence. If you really believe in something, then take strong, confident steps in that direction.

Say: "Divine Healing Intelligence, I ask you to release any self-doubt, confusion, weakness, indecision, and fear out of my heels, as well as all points of view, all patterns, and the positive and negative charges that contribute to this condition." Repeat the word "CLEAR" until you feel a shift occur.

Take off your shoes and socks. Stand on the ground and focus on letting go of anything that is stuck in your heels. Imagine all that stuckness, pain, and negativity releasing and flowing from your heels into the ground, where it is transmuted.

Say: "Divine Healing Intelligence, please install feelings of self-belief, clarity, balance, and strength. Allow me to move forward with courage, creativity, and confidence. Bring synchronicity and flow into my life. Thank you."

Rub your hands together, then place them slightly apart. Visualize earthy colors like browns and greens as lights of energy between your hands. Place your hands on your heels. Allow them to receive the grounding, clarifying vibration of moving forward. Hold your hands on your heels for a few minutes.

Say: "Divine Healing Intelligence, please heal and regenerate my heels to their full strength, balance, and mobility."

Unhealthy emotions to work with (page 171): Low Self-Esteem 190, Stress 194, Fear 179

Healthy emotions to work with (page 197): Confidence 198, Clarity 197, Respect 205

Colors to work with (page 211): Brown 212, Green 213, Pink 217

## Hips

### Possible Contributing Factors

Family problems and disagreements. Feeling used, unappreciated, angry, betrayed, deceived, let down, shot down, alienated. Experiencing strain, frustration, guilt, lack of support, too much responsibility. Feeling unacknowledged, taken advantage of, manipulated.

### Remedy

Who or what do you carry on your hips? Who are you taking responsibility for? Who are you supporting? Stand, and shake your hips. As you do this, imagine yourself shaking out old family beliefs and programming. If you have difficulty shaking your hips, then massage them in a circular motion with your hands.

Close your eyes and imagine a recycling bin in front of you that transmutes all dense and negative energy. Using your hands, remove all the stuck negativity from your hips—fear, frustration, guilt, and old family programming—and place this energy in the bin, where it will be dissolved. You may sense yourself pulling out heavy energy or you may see images, such as grayness, smoke, knives, or even people, coming out of your hips.

Say: "Divine Healing Intelligence, I ask you to release all the family problems, disagreements, conflicting emotions, guilt, sadness, grief, anger, and betrayal from my hips, as well as all points of view, the positive and negative charges, and all patterns that contribute to this condition." Repeat the word "CLEAR" until you feel a shift occur.

If you can, put on some music and shake your hips as if you are belly dancing. Feel the freedom of this experience. The more balanced and flexible your hips are, the more balanced, flexible, and creative your life will be.

Say: "Divine Healing Intelligence, please install feelings of peace, clarity, fulfillment, appreciation, relaxation, and serenity. Allow me to experience harmony, unity, and support in my life and in my family. Thank you."

Say: "Divine Healing Intelligence, please heal and regenerate my hips to their full strength, balance, and mobility."

Unhealthy emotions to work with (page 171): Criticism 175, Judgment 188, Frustration 181, Stuckness 196

Healthy emotions to work with (page 197): Clarity 197, Peace 204, Satisfaction 206, Recognition 204

Colors to work with (page 211): Orange 216, Green 213, Silver 219

## Hypothalamus

### Possible Contributing Factors

Feeling unbalanced, stressed, anxious, hormonal, emotional. Experiencing a disconnection from your Divine, spiritual Self. Confused and frustrated about the future and your role in life.

## Remedy

Say: "Divine Healing Intelligence, I ask you to release all mental and emotional imbalance, stress, fear, disconnection from the Divine, confusion, and frustration from my hypothalamus, as well as all points of view, all patterns, and the positive and negative charges that contribute to this condition." Repeat the word "CLEAR" until you feel a shift occur.

Say: "Divine Healing Intelligence, please help me find emotional, mental, and spiritual balance and a sense of well-being. Allow me to open my mind to a new, happier, and more positive vision of the future. Thank you."

Visualize your hypothalamus being filled with sparkling, golden light that activates and revitalizes it.

Say: "Divine Healing Intelligence, please heal and regenerate my hypothalamus and surrounding brain to their maximum health, vitality, and well-being."

*See also* Brain.

Unhealthy emotions to work with (page 171): Stress 194, Fear 179, Frustration 181
Healthy emotions to work with (page 197): Relaxation 205, Peace 204, Clarity 197
Colors to work with (page 211): Gold 213, Yellow 221, White 220

## Immune System

### Possible Contributing Factors

Insecurity, inner conflict, self-neglect, stress. Feeling pressured, threatened, manipulated, and with your guard down. Allowing people to take advantage of you. Too focused on the outside world. Pushing instead of allowing. Feeling like your integrity is being compromised. Not knowing how to say no. Feeling neglected and unloved. Thinking, *What is the point of this?* Feeling like you are struggling and not getting what you want. Overloading yourself.

### Remedy

Close your eyes. Become aware of all the problems you are carrying on your back, in your chest, and in your body. As you take a breath in, recognize a problem. As you breathe out, give yourself permission to let go of the tension you carry related to this problem. Ask for a Divine Solution. Do this several times until you feel freer.

Say: "Divine Healing Intelligence, I ask you to release all stress, insecurity, conflict, manipulation, resistance, frustration, and self-neglect from my immune system, as well as all points of view, all patterns, and the positive and negative charges that contribute to this condition." Repeat the word "CLEAR" until you feel a shift occur.

Shake your body of all its stress, suppression, and tension. Do this vigorously for thirty seconds then rest for fifteen seconds, breathing slowly and deeply. Repeat this process three or four times. To make it more fun, put on some funky music and shake your body to it.

Say: "Divine Healing Intelligence, please install feelings of security, stability, clarity, ease, and joy. Give me the courage to live my life the way I would love. Thank you."

To improve your immune system, place your ring finger and little finger on the tip of your thumb, extending the two remaining fingers away from the thumb. Hold this position between five and fifteen minutes. If your immune system is really down, you may like to practice this process three times a day.

Say: "Divine Healing Intelligence, please heal and regenerate my immune system to its maximum health, vibrancy, and well-being."

*See also* Thymus.


Unhealthy emotions to work with (page 171): Stress 194, Guilt 184, Frustration 181, Rejection 191

Healthy emotions to work with (page 197): Peace 204, Forgiveness 200, Relaxation 205, Joy 203

Colors to work with (page 211): Green 213, Blue 211, Orange 216, Purple 217


## Jaw

### Possible Contributing Factors

Holding tension, stress, suppression. Difficulty communicating how you feel. Judgment, criticism, fear. Inability to stand up for yourself and ask for what you want.

Guilt, blame, faultfinding. Feeling locked in. Holding on to anger and resentment. Stuck in a pattern without knowing how to break free and move forward.

## Remedy

Rub your hands together. Then hold them slightly apart. Visualize two balls of orange light in your hands. Place your palms on your jaw. Gently move your hands in a circular motion on either side of your jaw while breathing deeply and slowly. Focus on allowing this orange light to melt the tension inside your jaw. Do this for two to three minutes.

Say: "Divine Healing Intelligence, please help me to release all stress, tension, suppression, judgment, criticism, limitation, and fear from my jaw, as well as all points of view, all patterns, and the positive and negative charges that contribute to this condition." Repeat the word "CLEAR" until you feel a shift occur.

Focus on completely relaxing your fingers, toes, neck, head, and jaw. Allow your body to soften and let go. Place the tip of your tongue on the roof of your mouth. Breathe slowly and deeply. Focus on something positive as you allow yourself to smile internally. Then smile with your mouth, knowing that Divine Intelligence is on your side, assisting you to move through all your challenges.

Say: "Divine Healing Intelligence, please help me communicate with people in a way that they can hear and understand what I am saying. Give me the confidence to ask for what I want, and to become more creative and spontaneous in my life. Thank you."

To strengthen your jaw, bend your middle finger and press your thumb over it. Extend the rest of your fingers. Hold this position for three to five minutes while taking in deep, slow breaths. Make sure your jaw is relaxed.

Say: "Divine Healing Intelligence, please heal, relax, and regenerate my jaw and all related organs to their maximum health, vitality, and well-being."

Unhealthy emotions to work with (page 171): Stress 194, Anger 173, Guilt 184, Fear 179, Stuckness 196, Judgment 188

Healthy emotions to work with (page 197): Relaxation 205, Peace 204, Forgiveness 200, Love 203

Colors to work with (page 211): Silver 219, Orange 216, Green 213, Pink 217

## Joints

### Possible Contributing Factors

Suppressing or pushing down pain from the past, especially guilt, resentment, and anger. Holding on to the belief that there is not enough for you: not enough money, love, happiness, joy, opportunities, and so on. Feeling stuck. Critical of yourself and others. Impeded movement.

### Remedy

Close your eyes. Focus on any joints that are giving you problems. Ask yourself:

*What is blocking me from being flexible or allowing myself to move forward?*
*Where am I buying into other people's beliefs in limitation and lack?*

Allow yourself to receive a response. The more you can relax and breathe while asking questions, the clearer the response will be. You may need to change your mind about lack and limitation, and learn more about flexibility and flow.

Say: "Divine Healing Intelligence, I ask you to release all blockages, limitations, beliefs in lack, suppressed emotions, and feelings of guilt and anger from my joints, as well as all points of view, all patterns, and the positive and negative charges that contribute to this condition." Repeat the word "CLEAR" until you feel a shift occur.

Imagine that you have a little flask in your hands that contains healing oil. Pour that oil on the joint. Observe as the healing oil moves into the joint to create more ease and flexibility. Imagine what it would be like to move that joint without pain or discomfort. Then move it and become aware of the difference.

Say: "Divine Healing Intelligence, please install feelings of flexibility; movement; and flow of love, happiness, and joy. Allow me to move forward with ease and grace. Thank you."

Say: "Divine Healing Intelligence, please heal and regenerate my joints to their maximum strength, flexibility, and well-being."

Unhealthy emotions to work with (page 171): Guilt 184, Anger 173, Stuckness 196, Criticism 175

Healthy emotions to work with (page 197): Forgiveness 200, Peace 204, Respect 205, Support 206

Colors to work with (page 211): Green 213, Pink 217, Orange 216

## Kidneys

### Possible Contributing Factors

Living with guilt, regret, resentment, blame, ancient sadness. Holding on to destructive beliefs and memories from the past. Suffering with a limited, short-term memory because all attention is stuck in the past. Exhaustion, depression, numbness, paralyzing fear. Focusing on the negative aspects of life, unable to trust, difficulty dealing with challenging situations. Crumbling under pressure. Giving up.

### Remedy

Rub your hands together, then hold them slightly apart. Visualize two balls of green energy in your hands. Allow the energy to grow stronger.

Say: "Divine Healing Intelligence, please activate my healing abilities and allow green healing light to flow from my hands into my kidneys."

Place your hands on your back, just above your kidneys. Breathe in the green energy. As you take deep breaths, focus on distributing this green light into your arms and hands to assist the healing energy to flow more powerfully into your kidneys.

Say: "Divine Healing Intelligence, please help me to release all guilt, numbness, resentment, negativity, distrust, and regret from my kidneys, as well as all points of view, all patterns, and the positive and negative charges that contribute to this condition." Repeat the word "CLEAR" until you feel a shift occur.

Using your index and middle fingers, tap gently and slowly underneath your eyes, starting on the outside and moving toward your nose, then out again. Do this for thirty seconds, while taking deep, slow breaths in and out. Not only will it help you to cleanse your kidneys, but it will also to get rid of your under-eye bags and puffiness.

Say: "Divine Healing Intelligence, please help me take responsibility for my life, forgive myself for past mistakes, and move forward with renewed confidence and positivity. Thank you."

Say: "Divine Healing Intelligence, please heal, regenerate, and revitalize my kidneys and all related organs to their maximum health, vitality, and well-being."

Unhealthy emotions to work with (page 171): Sadness 193, Anger 173, Guilt 184, Fear 179

Healthy emotions to work with (page 197): Forgiveness 200, Innocence 202, Honor 202, Joy 203

Colors to work with (page 211): Orange 216, Silver 219, Green 214

## Knees

### Possible Contributing Factors

Control, blame, judgment, anger, resentment, frustration, inflexibility. Feeling stuck. Difficulty dealing with a person, issue, or situation from the past. Confusion. Frozen desires and unfulfilled dreams. Unresolved family issues. Difficulty making decisions and keeping commitments. Fear of moving forward. A great need to know what will happen next.

### Right Knee

Issues with a significant male in your life: father, brother, uncle, and so on. Difficulty moving forward in your career. Limited thinking. Fear of failure. Asking yourself, *Where am I inflexible in my life?*

### Left Knee

Issues with a mother, sister, aunt, or significant female in your life. Holding on to sadness, hurt, and loss from the past. Feeling like a victim. Constant criticism. Holding yourself back.

## Remedy

Stand. Ask yourself:

*Am I willing to let go of controlling, blaming, and judging myself and others?*
*Can I give myself permission to move forward with trust, love, and certainty?*

If the answer is yes, visualize releasing all the fear, blame, and inflexibility. You may imagine cutting yourself free from heavy ropes of control, or taking rocks of fear out of various parts of your body and throwing them into the ocean.

Say: "Divine Healing Intelligence, I ask you to release all blame, judgment, fear, anger, confusion, hurt, loss, sadness, and inflexibility from my knees, as well as all points of view, all patterns, and the positive and negative charges that contribute to this condition." Repeat the word "CLEAR" until you feel a shift occur.

Ask yourself: *What possibilities are now available to me?* Imagine a life of infinite options, flexibility, flow, and satisfaction. Now, take a step forward. Allow yourself to really live this experience of freedom, empowerment, and flow in the moment. Breathe deeply and really savor the experience of expansion.

Say: "Divine Healing Intelligence, please install deeper awareness, flexibility, certainty, and a sense of freedom. Allow me to take responsibility for my actions, and to open myself up to incredible new opportunities and ways of experiencing life. Thank you."

Now, sit down and rub your hands. Feel the heat and tingling sensation in your hands, and then visualize a powerful green ray of light emanating from them. Place your hands on your knees and sense this green ray as it moves through your knees, releasing all their stuckness and density, and regenerating them. Keep your hands on your knees until you feel the process has concluded.

Say: "Divine Healing Intelligence, please heal and regenerate my knees to their maximum strength, flexibility, and well-being."

Unhealthy emotions to work with (page 171): Anger 173, Control 174, Criticism
    175, Resentment 192, Stuckness 196
Healthy emotions to work with (page 197): Flexibility and Movement 200,
    Encouragement 199, Confidence 198, Peace 204, Forgiveness 200
Colors to work with (page 211): Green 213, Pink 217, Orange 216

## Large Intestine

### Possible Contributing Factors

Crying spells, confusion, irritation, frustration, stagnation, and anger. Thinking that you can't do anything right. Wanting to run away and hide from the world. Feeling that you are too different and that no one understands you. Difficulty seeing other people's points of view. Dogmatically defending your position in arguments. Extremely sensitive, thin-skinned.

### Remedy

Say: "Divine Healing Intelligence, I ask you to release all hurt, irritation, frustration, confusion, and stagnation from my large intestine, as well as all points of view, all patterns, and the positive and negative charges that contribute to this condition." Repeat the word "CLEAR" until you feel a shift occur.

Say: "Divine Healing Intelligence, please support my ability to follow through my ideas to completion. Allow me to become more open-minded and flexible, and to embrace everyone's individuality and creativity. Thank you."

Say: "Divine Healing Intelligence, please heal, regenerate, and revitalize my large intestine and all related organs to their maximum health, vitality, and well-being."

*See also* Bowels.

Unhealthy emotions to work with (page 171): Stress 194, Frustration 181, Anger 173, Judgment 188

Healthy emotions to work with (page 197): Freedom 201, Encouragement 199, Happiness 201

Colors to work with (page 211): Orange 216, Yellow 221, Brown 212, Blue 211

## *Legs*

### Possible Contributing Factors

Feeling overwhelmed by the pressure, strain, and demands of your life. Frightened by perceived obstacles. Carrying a heavy load of unresolved issues from the past that weigh you down. Feeling unsupported, and buying into self-doubt and insecurity.

### *Right Leg*

Difficulty taking action. Feeling undermined, restricted, insecure, unsupported, unsteady. Moving in the wrong direction, sabotaging yourself, resisting the flow of life. Not giving yourself enough time to tune in and become clear about your purpose.

### *Left Leg*

Feeling hurt, angry, oversensitive, self-critical, pressured, worried. Being held back by unresolved issues from your past. Fear of moving forward and taking responsibility for your actions. Overly concerned about what other people will think about your choices. Doing things you dislike because you seek approval or need money to survive.

### Remedy

Thank your legs for carrying you. Take a good look at them. Appreciate them. Think of all the wonderful things your legs allow you to do: stand, walk, run, jump, dance, drive, move. What are they worth to you? Would you sell them for a million dollars? Not likely. Realize that your legs are priceless. You are already abundant.

Become aware of how your legs feel. Do they feel bound, heavy, and weak; or light, free, and strong? If they feel bound, limited, and burdened, ask the Divine Healing Intelligence to help you release these burdens and limitations.

Say: "Divine Healing Intelligence, I ask you to release all burdens, obstacles, limitations, heaviness, hurt, anger, pressure, fear, and weakness from my legs, as well as all points of view, all patterns, and the positive and negative charges that contribute to this condition." Repeat the word "CLEAR" until you feel a shift occur.

Focus on all the pressure and stuckness you carry in your legs. Shake them out. You can do this by standing and shaking your legs one at a time, or by sitting and shaking them together. If you can't stand up, shake them while sitting down. Shake for thirty seconds then relax for thirty seconds, and feel the energy tingling in your legs. Repeat the process several times. Then march or tap your feet for sixty seconds and relax for thirty seconds. Repeat this process several times. Dance around to music. You will stimulate the circulation in your legs.

Breathe deeply. Focus on the warmth and tingling in your legs, and intensify it. Using the power of your mind, direct the warmth and tingling to move around your legs. Make the energy warm for thirty seconds, and then cool it for thirty seconds. Continue this process for five minutes. You can create warmth by focusing on the colors red and orange, and coolness by focusing on blue and turquoise.

Move your hands along your legs, gently caressing them from your ankles to the top of your thighs. Imagine that your fingers are like the hairs of two big paintbrushes and that you are painting your legs the color pink. If you become aware of any density, allow the pink color to flow over it, dissipating it.

Say: "Divine Healing Intelligence, please increase my confidence, clarity, self-empowerment, and creativity. Allow me to experience ease, flow, and balance in my life. Give me the strength to follow my dreams with total support from people around me. Thank you."

Massage your legs and focus on moving forward, feeling confident and clear in what you desire to experience in your life. Imagine your legs moving with ease and grace. Then stand and walk confidently.

If you have problems with circulation, you may want to take a soft bristle brush and scrub your legs vigorously for thirty seconds (don't do this if you have any skin irritations). Then rest for twenty seconds. Repeat this process three to five times.

Say: "Divine Healing Intelligence, please heal and regenerate my legs, knees, and ankles to their full health, vitality, and flexibility."

Unhealthy emotions to work with (page 171): Stress 194, Fear 179, Anger 173, Feeling Overwhelmed 180

Healthy emotions to work with (page 197): Flexibility and Movement 200, Clarity 197, Confidence 198, Success 207

Colors to work with (page 211): Red 218, Orange 216, Blue 211, Turquoise 219, Pink 217

## *Liver*

### Possible Contributing Factors

Irrational frustration, aggression, rage, guilt, fear. Desire to inflict self-punishment and sabotage your progress. Constant inner struggle and conflict. Difficulty making decisions. Often finding fault or blame with others. Inclined to act like a victim, with a "poor me" attitude. Overlooking other people's advice and suggestions. Difficulty forgiving and letting go. Trouble sleeping, relaxing, and trusting.

### Remedy

Rub your hands together, then place them slightly apart. Imagine that you have a ball of green and yellow energy in your hands. Place your hands on your liver while visualizing or sensing this ball of energy moving inside it and purifying it, removing damaged tissue, infection, toxins, anger, fear, frustration, and any other negative feelings.

Say: "Divine Healing Intelligence, I ask you to release all irrational frustration, aggression, rage, fear, indecision, guilt, and blame from my liver, as well as all points of view, all patterns, and the positive and negative charges that contribute to this condition." Repeat the word "CLEAR" until you feel a shift occur.

Press your fingers together. Place your hands on your liver and rub this area in a circular motion clockwise three to five times. Then tap the liver area.

Say: "Divine Healing Intelligence, please increase my levels of peace, patience, and harmony. Allow me to see that things are perfect as they are, and that all I have to do to enjoy my life is to slow down, become aware of all the wonderful things life offers, and just take one step at a time."

Find the deepest hollow of the cheeks, where the jawbone connects to the cheekbones. Place your index and middle fingers there, and massage vigorously for thirty seconds. Then rest for twenty seconds. Repeat four times.

Say: "Divine Healing Intelligence, please heal and regenerate my liver and all related organs to their full health, vitality, and flexibility."

Unhealthy emotions to work with (page 171): Stress 194, Fear 179, Frustration 181, Anger 173, Guilt 184

Healthy emotions to work with (page 197): Peace 204, Forgiveness 200, Love 203, Respect 205, Compassion 198

Colors to work with (page 211): Green 213, Yellow 221

## Lungs

### Possible Contributing Factors

Sad, yearning, weepy, anguished, tired, suppressed. Difficulty expressing or standing up for yourself. Propensity to put other people's needs and desires first, and to overdo things until you run out of breath. Inability to say no. Feeling smothered or overprotected. Difficulty being independent. Confused or cloudy thinking. Constant need for encouragement and support.

### Remedy

Rub your hands together, then place them slightly apart. Visualize orange rays of light in your palms. Place your hands on your lungs, and breathe in the orange light. Allow it to warm your lungs, and cleanse and dissipate the toxicity.

Say: "Divine Healing Intelligence, I ask you to release all feelings of sadness, anguish, suppression, dependence, and tiredness from my lungs. Help me let go of my tendency to put myself last and to do too much for others; my inability to say no; as well as all points of view, all patterns, and the positive and negative charges that contribute to this condition." Repeat the word "CLEAR" until you feel a shift occur.

Place your middle and index fingers on the outer edge of your lips. Press inward as strongly as you can handle and rotate in a circular motion, first clockwise for thirty seconds and then counterclockwise for another thirty seconds. Then relax for twenty seconds. Repeat this process four times.

Tilt your head back slightly as you take a slow, deep breath in, and then tilt slightly forward as you breathe out. As you breathe in, visualize healing green light moving into your lungs and regenerating them. As you breathe out, visualize any density or toxicity releasing. Do this for two or three minutes.

Say: "Divine Healing Intelligence, please intensify my ability to express myself fully, creatively, and confidently. Allow me to value and honor myself, and to become independent. Thank you."

Say: "Divine Healing Intelligence, please heal and regenerate my lungs and all related organs to their full health, vitality, and flexibility."

*See also* Chest.

Unhealthy emotions to work with (page 171): Sadness 193, Frustration 181, Low
    Self-Esteem 190, Feeling Overwhelmed 180
Healthy emotions to work with (page 197): Peace 204, Joy 203, Freedom 201,
    Relaxation 205
Colors to work with (page 211): Orange 216, Green 213, Pink 217, Magenta 215

## *Mouth*

### Possible Contributing Factors

Lack of understanding, closed mind, limited ideas. Having a bad attitude, saying things that are hurtful to others, criticizing, judging, spreading rumors, gossiping.

Worrying too much and not loving or nurturing yourself enough. Eating unhealthy food. Self-hatred.

## Remedy

Focus on your mouth. How does it feel inside? Become aware of your tongue, your teeth, your lips. What is the taste inside your mouth? Is it fresh or stale? Are you able to chew and digest what life presents you, or are you resisting and saying no to life? In what condition are your teeth? Are they strong, or are they rotting and loosening? What does your mouth want to share with you?

Relax your mouth. Become aware of the role it plays in your life. It helps you eat, taste, digest, talk, connect with others, and express affection.

When you eat, focus on chewing your food properly to help with the digestive process. When you talk to people, focus on expressing what you really desire to say. When you show affection, be aware of the feelings you are showing.

Say: "Divine Healing Intelligence, I ask you to release all the close-mindedness, limitation, bad attitude, judgment, and criticism that comes out of my mouth, as well as all points of view, all patterns, and the positive and negative charges that contribute to this condition." Repeat the word "CLEAR" until you feel a shift occur.

Close your eyes, and imagine breathing in the clearest white light through your mouth. Hold your breath for a moment and imagine this white energy swishing through your mouth as if it were mouthwash. Allow it to move throughout your mouth, dissipating and releasing all the density, tightness, and stress, and then spit it all out. Repeat the process three to four times. You can also use other colors, like pink, orange, and blue.

Say: "Divine Healing Intelligence, please allow me to become more understanding, generous, and positive. Help me to have a better attitude about my life and the people I spend time with. Thank you."

Say: "Divine Healing Intelligence, please heal and regenerate my mouth, tongue, and teeth to their full health, vitality, and flexibility."

Unhealthy emotions to work with (page 171): Worry 197, Criticism 175, Judgment 188

Healthy emotions to work with (page 197): Honor 202, Compassion 198,
  Forgiveness 200
Colors to work with (page 211): White 220, Pink 217, Orange 216, Blue 211

## Muscles

### Possible Contributing Factors

Stress, worry. Holding on to fear, anger, sadness. Feeling overwhelmed and that you need to control your life. Thinking and tensing up rather than feeling and letting go. Being a workaholic and feeling the weight of responsibilities you carry. Difficulty expressing your true feelings for fear of not being accepted. Stuck in fight-or-flight response. Frozen inside.

### Remedy

Focus on your muscles. Take a deep breath in, and then tense your muscles. Hold the tension for ten counts while holding your breath. Then relax your muscles and slowly breathe out. Repeat this process several times.

Say: "Divine Healing Intelligence, I ask you to release all tension, worry, fear, stress, anger, sadness, and overwhelming feelings from my muscles, as well as all points of view, all patterns, and the positive and negative charges that contribute to this condition." Repeat the word "CLEAR" until you feel a shift occur.

As you breathe in, imagine filling your muscles with healing blue light. Allow the blue light to dissolve all the tension, stuckness, and density from your muscles.

Say: "Divine Healing Intelligence, please help me relax and become more open-minded and wise. Give me the courage to deal with my emotions, and free myself from all negativity and dense energy that I carry. Thank you."

Say: "Divine Healing Intelligence, please heal and regenerate my muscles to their full health, strength, and flexibility."

Unhealthy emotions to work with (page 171): Stress 194, Fear 179, Anger 173,
  Feeling Overwhelmed 180

Healthy emotions to work with (page 197): Relaxation 205, Faith 199, Satisfaction 206

Colors to work with (page 211): Orange 216, Green 213, Blue 211

## Nails

### Possible Contributing Factors

Difficulty dealing with mundane, everyday challenges. Pesky, annoying, irritating beliefs, thoughts, experiences that lodge in and get stuck. A sense of stagnation or the feeling of pushing against a wall. Recurring stresses and worries, which feel like a waste of time but take up too much of it. Upset or irritation with a close friend, family member, or partner. Feeling stressed out and overwhelmed, as if someone is pushing past your protective barriers.

### Remedy

Become aware of who or what is getting under your nails. Who are you not dealing with? What is irritating you? Rather than pushing emotions under the carpet, you need to learn how to deal with them. The first step is to admit what you are feeling.

Focus on the affected nail. Become aware of the emotion stored there, and, using the fingers of your other hand, imagine that you are pulling this emotion out. As you extract each emotion out of your nail, say it out loud: "Fear," "Anger," "Blame," and so on. Then place the negative emotion into a red fire, and observe its dissipation until the flame changes from red to white or red to green. Imagine painting your nail in a clear, healing, regenerative liquid.

Say: "Divine Healing Intelligence, I ask you to release all the ways I feel unprotected, overwhelmed, stuck, and unable to deal with my thoughts and feelings, as well as all points of view, all patterns, and the positive and negative charges that contribute to this condition." Repeat the word "CLEAR" until you feel a shift occur.

Say: "Divine Healing Intelligence, please help me to handle life and all its challenges in an empowered, positive, and healthy way. Give me the right words to express myself clearly, gently, and skillfully so that people will truly hear and understand. Thank you."

Say: "Divine Healing Intelligence, please heal and regenerate my nails to their full health, strength, and well-being."

Unhealthy emotions to work with (page 171): Irritation 187, Frustration 181, Worry 197, Stress 194
Healthy emotions to work with (page 197): Peace 204, Support 206, Clarity 197
Colors to work with (page 211): Red 218, White 220, Green 213

## *Neck*

### Possible Contributing Factors

Relationship problems. Inability to communicate feelings. Difficulty making commitments. Feeling stuck, inflexible, pressured, like something or someone is strangling you. Propensity to sweep issues under the carpet so you don't have to deal with them. Holding on to unresolved issues in relationships, especially with parents, children, or past partners. Often seeing yourself in a negative self-image. Spending too much time thinking and trying to work things out, and not enough time being aware of your feelings by tuning into your intuition.

### Remedy

Have you been saying that someone or something is a pain in the neck? Are your commitments strangling you? Where in your life are you unwilling to bend and be flexible? Is there someone you need to talk to?

Focus on your breathing. Allow your shoulder to drop and your neck to relax. Focus on allowing the muscles to loosen. Tune into your neck by placing your hands gently on it. Breathe in to that area and ask yourself questions, such as:

*If there were a thought stored in my neck, what would it be?*
*If there were an emotion stored in my neck, what would it be?*
*If there were a picture or a memory stored in my neck, what would it be?*
*What do I need to change to feel better?*

Wait for a response, and acknowledge it or write it down.

Close your eyes. Imagine taking ropes, chains, tightness, density, and inflexibility out of your neck. Place it all into a rainbow flame and watch it burn.

Say: "Divine Healing Intelligence, please delete and dissolve all the ways I am inflexible, stressed, fearful, and uptight. Please draw out all pain from my neck, all beliefs that someone or something is causing me pain, as well as all points of view, all patterns, and the positive and negative charges that contribute to this condition." Repeat the word "CLEAR" until you feel a shift occur.

Now, bathe your neck with healing rays of green light. Imagine that this green light is circling your neck, releasing density, relaxing the muscles, and healing pain.

Say: "Divine Healing Intelligence, please install flexibility, awareness, patience, trust, faith, and openness to new possibilities in my life. Help me resolve issues from my past and move forward with clarity into the future. Thank you."

Say: "Divine Healing Intelligence, please unwind, relax, and loosen my neck."

Unhealthy emotions to work with (page 171): Stuckness 196, Fear 179, Stress 194

Healthy emotions to work with (page 197): Flexibility and Movement 200, Forgiveness 200, Honor 202, Respect 205

Colors to work with (page 211): Green 213, Blue 211

## Nervous System

### Possible Contributing Factors

Hitting a raw nerve. Feeling attacked or under threat. Holding on to shame, guilt, embarrassment. Constricting the nervous system by worrying about the future or being stuck in the past. Pushing, straining, fighting, struggling. Feeling nervy, edgy, tense, anxious. Experiencing a lack of balance, rest, and relaxation. Overworked, over-committed, and pushed to the limit. Looking for an adrenaline rush or some kind of excitement. Prone to addictions, such as cigarettes or other drugs.

## Remedy

Sit. Place your hands on your thighs, and open the palms of your hands so that they are facing upwards. Close your eyes. Focus on your shoulders, neck, and back. Take a few deep breaths in and allow your shoulders to relax. Take another deep breath in, and visualize a blue ray streaming down into your head and down your back, bathing your whole nervous system in light. As you breathe out, imagine all the nervous tension, density, and stress leaving your body. Repeat this process eight to ten times.

Say: "Divine Healing Intelligence, please help me regenerate my nervous system by letting go of feelings of judgment, or of being attacked or threatened. Please help me to delete and dissolve all the shame, guilt, worry, and embarrassment I carry in my nervous system, as well as all points of view, all patterns, and the positive and negative charges that contribute to this condition." Repeat the word "CLEAR" until you feel a shift occur.

Extend your index and middle fingers of both hands. Place the ring fingers and little fingers on top of your thumb. As you hold this gesture, close your eyes and take slow, deep breaths for five to fifteen minutes, allowing your body to relax. You may also like to play some soothing music. Focus on something pleasant that makes you feel calm. Visualize the green light bathing and regenerating your whole spine and nervous system. You might imagine yourself floating in a beautiful blue ocean or relaxing on a beach, allowing the warmth of the sun to dissolve all tension. Or you can imagine your perfect day: how it would begin, who you would meet, what you would do, and how you would feel.

Say: "Divine Healing Intelligence, please assist me in effortlessly letting go of all my tension and install peace, clarity, serenity, and relaxation into my nervous system. Thank you."

Say: "Divine Healing Intelligence, please unwind, relax, and regenerate my nervous system to its maximum health, vitality, and well-being."

Unhealthy emotions to work with (page 171): Attack 174, Shame 193, Guilt 184, Feeling Overwhelmed 180, Stress 194

Healthy emotions to work with (page 197): Respect 205, Support 206, Clarity 197, Relaxation 205, Freedom 201

Colors to work with (page 211): Blue 211, Green 213, Gold 213, White 220

## *Nose*

### Possible Contributing Factors

Looking for love and attention. Not listening to your intuition. Feeling unnoticed, invisible, unimportant, unworthy. Feeling tired, run-down, overwhelmed. Propensity to interfere with other people's affairs. Being nosy, gossipy, judgmental, and hurtful.

### Remedy

Gently place your hand on top of your nose. How does it feel? Is it easy to breathe through your nose, or are there blockages and irritation?

When people have blocked sinuses, they often feel run-down and want to keep others away. How do you feel about the people around you? Many animals use their sense of smell as an intuitive mechanism. How open are you to developing your intuition and following your nose, even if it shows you what you are not expecting or wanting to see or experience? What insights does your nose want to share with you?

Say: "Divine Healing Intelligence, I ask you to release all the ways I don't listen to my intuition and feel overwhelmed, unimportant, invisible, and unworthy. Please help me to let go of all the tiredness and constriction from my nose, as well as all points of view, all patterns, and the positive and negative charges that contribute to this condition." Repeat the word "CLEAR" until you feel a shift occur.

To help clear your sinuses, bring together the tips of your thumb, index, and middle fingers. Bend the other two fingers and place them on your palm. Do the same with the other hand, and then place both positioned hands at the level of your stomach. Hold this gesture for five to ten minutes, three to four times a day.

Say: "Divine Healing Intelligence, please help me to connect to my intuition and to Divine Wisdom. Teach me to value myself highly and to feel worthy of new, wonderful opportunities that I am attracting into my life. Thank you."

Close your eyes. Imagine a ray of indigo light moving through your sinuses and dissolving any buildup of mucus or other density. Focus on slowly breathing in the clean air through your sinuses. Allow yourself to enjoy the experience.

Say: "Divine Healing Intelligence, please clear, heal, and regenerate my nose to its maximum health, vitality, and well-being."

Unhealthy emotions to work with (page 171): Judgment 188, Criticism 175, Feeling Overwhelmed 180

Healthy emotions to work with (page 197): Love 203, Recognition 204, Respect 205, Honor 202

Colors to work with (page 211): Indigo 214, Purple 217, Violet 220

## Esophagus

### Possible Contributing Factors

Swallowing grief, anger, and hurt. Difficulty asking for what you need or desire. Thinking that you are second best. Believing that what you have to say is not important.

### Remedy

Picture your esophagus; tune into it. Does it look clear and healthy, or is there heavy, dense, or stuck energy there?

You need to start expressing your feelings and valuing yourself. With whom are you angry, upset, or hurt? Imagine this person or a group of people in front of you. Say out loud what it is that you want them to know. You may start by saying something like: "Dear [insert the name of the person or experience that has kept you stuck], I want you to know that [state whatever it is that you need to express]." Express it fully without holding back. Once you have verbalized it, you will become clear on what you have been holding on to and what you need to express.

Say: "Divine Healing Intelligence, I ask you to melt the deep-seated sadness, grief, anger, hurt, feelings of inferiority, and stuckness out of my esophagus, as well as all points of view, all patterns, and the positive and negative charges that contribute to this condition." Repeat the word "CLEAR" until you feel a shift occur.

Visualize an orange ray of light moving through your entire esophagus and dissolving all density, degeneration, and limitation.

Say: "Divine Healing Intelligence, please intensify my ability to breathe easily; communicate clearly; value myself highly; and express myself fully, lovingly, and courageously. Thank you."

Allow the orange ray to spin like a wheel of orange light, regenerating your esophagus.

Say: "Divine Healing Intelligence, please heal and regenerate my esophagus and all related organs to their maximum health, vitality, and well-being. Thank you."

Unhealthy emotions to work with (page 171): Sadness 193, Frustration 181, Low
    Self-Esteem 190, Feeling Overwhelmed 180
Healthy emotions to work with (page 197): Forgiveness 200, Compassion 198,
    Encouragement 199
Colors to work with (page 211): Orange 216, Green 213, Blue 211

## Ovaries

### Possible Contributing Factors

Holding on to old hurts, especially from men. Invalidating yourself. Not trusting your intuition. Low self-esteem, and feelings of neglect and victimhood. Rejection of your femininity or feminine nature. Carrying a belief that to be feminine is to be weak. Propensity to worry about everyone and everything. Focusing on aging: the loss of power, beauty, and appeal. Not allowing yourself to enjoy your sensuality and womanhood. In some cases, issues with fertility.

### Remedy

How do you feel about being female? Do you feel that you embrace your femininity and sensuality, or do you try to be a superwoman, doing everything for others and ignoring your own needs?

When buying or doing something for yourself, do you think, *Oh no, I could not possibly afford this for myself, but if my partner, child, friend, dog, cat, or car needed it, then I would definitely buy it without a second thought?*

Become aware of your own needs and desires. What wonderful things do you deserve to have in your life? If you can't have them now, then when can you? If you don't look after and give to yourself, who will look out for your needs and desires?

Allow yourself to enjoy your femininity, your sensuality, your body. What clothes make you feel feminine and beautiful? Buy and wear them. What words, images, feelings, or actions make you feel empowered? Think them, feel them, say them, do them. Allow yourself to enjoy being female. Realize that embracing your femininity is beautiful, courageous, and strong.

Say: "Divine Healing Intelligence, help me stop rejecting, invalidating, and neglecting myself, and taking myself for granted. Allow me to release all the ways I feel unworthy, weak, disempowered, and lost from my ovaries, as well as all points of view, all patterns, and the positive and negative charges that contribute to this condition." Repeat the word "CLEAR" until you feel a shift occur.

Place your hands on your lower abdomen over your ovaries. Focus on sending your ovaries your deepest, most intense love and appreciation. Thank them for all the wonderful work they do. If you have children or desire to have them, thank your ovaries for their gift of life. If you are still menstruating, thank them for connecting you to the moon's rhythm, the feminine cycle.

If you desire to have children but cannot, forgive your ovaries for being unable to fulfill your wishes. Ask the Divine Intelligence of the universe to support you in bringing children into your life in a different way so that you can still experience the joy of their company.

Surround your ovaries with a healing yellow sunlight. Allow this light to dissipate any density to penetrate deep into the ovaries, restoring their health and vitality.

Say: "Divine Healing Intelligence, please help me to value, honor, and listen to my intuition and Divine Guidance. Allow me to take pleasure in my femininity, sensuality, and physicality. Thank you."

Say: "Divine Healing Intelligence, please heal and regenerate my ovaries and all related organs to their maximum health, vitality, and well-being."

Unhealthy emotions to work with (page 171): Anger 173, Judgment 188, Sadness 193

Healthy emotions to work with (page 197): Forgiveness 200, Compassion 198,
    Honor 202
Colors to work with (page 211): Yellow 221, Orange 216, Gold 213

## Pancreas

### Possible Contributing Factors

Inability to savor the sweetness in life. Feeling smothered, over-mothered, or under-nurtured. Experiencing over-concern, hopelessness, helplessness, and lack of control. Easily affected by others. Low self-esteem, feelings of bitterness, confusion, unfairness, and unjustness. Craving sugar, sweetness, and softness. Often looking for quick fixes and then experiencing disappointment. Very gullible and easily swayed. Stubborn and immovable.

### Remedy

Place the middle fingers of both hands flat against each other and fold the other fingers together. Hold this gesture in front of your solar plexus for three to four minutes while taking deep, slow breaths.

Say: "Divine Healing Intelligence, help me to release any bitterness, over-concern, and feelings of helplessness, hopelessness, and confusion from my pancreas, as well as all points of view, all patterns, and the positive and negative charges that contribute to this condition." Repeat the word "CLEAR" until you feel a shift occur.

Close your eyes and focus on your pancreas. When you visualize your pancreas in your mind's eye, does it look clear and healthy or dark and heavy?

If it's dark and heavy, imagine holding a vacuum cleaner. Suck the dark, heavy spots from your pancreas until it clears of all impurity.

Rub your hands together for a minute. Place them slightly apart and visualize a bright orange ray of light between your palms. Place your hands on your pancreas, and sense the orange light moving deep inside, healing, regenerating, and revitalizing it. Repeat "Heal, clear, and regenerate now" several times for two minutes.

Say: "Divine Healing Intelligence, please help me experience sweetness, nurturing, and joy. Help me to become stronger, more confident, and more empowered so that I can be heard, listened to, and validated. Thank you."

Say: "Divine Healing Intelligence, please heal and regenerate my pancreas and all related organs to their maximum health, vitality, and well-being."

Unhealthy emotions to work with (page 171): Sadness 193, Hopelessness 186, Guilt 184, Control 174, Rejection 191
Healthy emotions to work with (page 197): Clarity 197, Confidence 198, Freedom 201, Joy 203
Colors to work with (page 211): Orange 216, Yellow 221

## *Penis*

### Possible Contributing Factors

Lack of belief in self; fear of intimacy; feelings of rejection, anger, guilt, victimization. Feeling hurt by someone that you love or once loved. Difficulty trusting others; feeling vulnerable, alone, scared, unlovable, depressed. Holding on to too many judgments and criticisms. Denying yourself pleasure and fun. Carrying many unresolved issues with family members—father, mother, brother, sister, wife, lover, children, and so on.

### Remedy

For whom do you carry feelings of hurt, guilt, anger, and resentment? What steps would you be willing to take to forgive these people and let go of your emotional blockages?

Visualize old guilt, fear, rejection, anger, and resentment releasing from your whole reproductive system like rings of gray smoke. Give yourself permission to move forward.

Visualize beautiful turquoise light entering your body, regenerating all the reproductive organs and restoring feelings of confidence, joy, pleasure, and connection. Give yourself permission to feel pleasure.

Say: "Divine Healing Intelligence, please help me release all feelings of rejection, anger, hurt, victimization, fear of intimacy, and isolation from my penis and reproductive system, as well as all points of view, all patterns, and the positive and negative charges that contribute to this condition." Repeat the word "CLEAR" until you feel a shift occur.

Say: "Divine Healing Intelligence, please help me forgive all the people who have hurt me, and bring back feelings of pleasure, sensuality, and empowerment, as well as experiences of intimacy and connection with others. Thank you."

Say: "Divine Healing Intelligence, please heal and regenerate my penis and all related organs to their maximum health, vitality, and well-being."

Unhealthy emotions to work with (page 171): Fear 179, Guilt 184, Anger 173, Resentment 192, Rejection 191
Healthy emotions to work with (page 197): Forgiveness 200, Innocence 202, Respect 205, Satisfaction 206
Colors to work with (page 211): Turquoise 219, Red 218, Green 213

## Pineal Gland

### Possible Contributing Factors

Feeling out of sync, dull, confused, unaware, disconnected, isolated. Going along with others and what they want rather than listening to your intuition. Ignorance, lack of awareness, skepticism, self-doubt, uncertainty, inflexibility, selfishness.

### Remedy

Close your eyes and focus on your pineal gland. Imagine that it is like a very small light globe in the middle of your brain. Visualize or sense this light globe being switched on, and allow it to light up your whole brain. When clear, the pineal gland can help you create a spiritual connection and receive inner wisdom.

Say: "Divine Healing Intelligence, please help me release all feelings of dullness, disconnection, isolation, ignorance, skepticism, and stubbornness from my pineal gland, as well as all points of view, all patterns, and the positive and negative charges that contribute to this condition." Repeat the word "CLEAR" until you feel a shift occur.

Say: "Divine Healing Intelligence, please help me to feel connected, open, and flexible. Give me a sense of balance, peace, and Divine Insight into my life. Thank you."

Say: "Divine Healing Intelligence, please heal and regenerate my pineal gland and all related glands to their maximum health, vitality, and well-being."

Unhealthy emotions to work with (page 171): Low Self-Esteem 190, Frustration 181, Feeling Overwhelmed 180
Healthy emotions to work with (page 197): Relaxation 205, Confidence 198, Peace 204, Joy 203
Colors to work with (page 211): Yellow 221, Indigo 214, Purple 217, White 220

## *Pituitary Gland*

### Possible Contributing Factors
Feeling depleted, suppressed, disheartened, hormonal, unemotional, confused. Experiencing sluggish memory, fear, instability. Feeling threatened. Difficulty making decisions. Constantly changing your mind.

### Remedy
Focus on your pituitary gland. Place your middle and index fingers of the left hand on your forehead, between your eyebrows, in the spot of the "third eye." Does it feel clear or dense? If it feels dense, relax your forehead and imagine using a purple flame of light (the color of the brow chakra) to dissolve all tension. You can also rub your hands together and create a purple flame between them. Then place your hands on or just above the pituitary gland with the intention of dissolving all tension. Next, gently rub and tap your middle finger on your forehead in between your eyebrows.

Say: "Divine Healing Intelligence, please help me release all tiredness, emotional instability, fear, and confusion from my pituitary gland, as well as all points of view, all patterns, and the positive and negative charges that contribute to this condition." Repeat the word "CLEAR" until you feel a shift occur.

Take deep breaths in and focus on your pituitary gland; as you breathe out, let go of any stress or pressure. Repeat this process three to five times.

Say: "Divine Healing Intelligence, please help me feel more energized, clear, vibrant, and full of life. Improve my memory and give me a sense of stability, security, and peace of mind. Thank you."

Using your left hand, massage your right thumb from base to tip as you focus on activating your pituitary gland. Surround the gland with violet light, and visualize or sense the healing energy regenerate your pituitary gland.

Say: "Divine Healing Intelligence, please heal and regenerate my pituitary gland and all related glands to their maximum health, vitality, and well-being."

Unhealthy emotions to work with (page 171): Fear 179, Depression 176, Low Self-Esteem 190

Healthy emotions to work with (page 197): Peace 204, Clarity 197, Love 203, Confidence 198

Colors to work with (page 211): Orange 216, Yellow 221, Indigo 214

## Prostate Gland

### Possible Contributing Factors
Feeling inferior, stuck, ashamed, suppressed, helpless, guarded. Lacking confidence, trust, and security. Rejecting your masculinity. Not sure how to express your feelings. Carrying deep-seated disappointment, resentment, and guilt.

### Remedy
How do you feel about yourself? Do you allow yourself to express your feelings, or do you suppress them? Do you feel you have been successful and achieved your life's goals, or do you carry feelings of failure?

Close your eyes and focus on your prostate. Imagine enveloping it with a green light. Ask what feelings, emotions, and experiences are stuck in your prostate gland. Imagine those feelings and experiences as weeds that you pull out of your prostate, then place the weeds into a fire and watch them burn.

Say: "Divine Healing Intelligence, please help me to release all stuckness; suppression; feelings of helplessness, inferiority, resentment, and shame; as well as all points of view, all patterns, and the positive and negative charges that contribute to this condition." Repeat the word "CLEAR" until you feel a shift occur.

Now, focus on feelings of confidence. If there were a color that could help you to feel confident, what would it be? Imagine pouring this color into your prostate. What thoughts or words make you feel confident? Say them out loud. Focus on an event or experience where you felt self-empowered and confident. Now, make that feeling stronger. Imagine pouring this feeling into your prostate gland as if it were liquid.

Say: "Divine Healing Intelligence, please increase my confidence and self-belief. Give me the courage to take positive action to create a life of happiness, fulfillment, and empowerment. Thank you."

Say: "Divine Healing Intelligence, please heal and regenerate my prostate gland and all related glands to their maximum health, vitality, and well-being."

Unhealthy emotions to work with (page 171): Stuckness 196, Shame 193, Hopelessness 186, Low Self-Esteem 190

Healthy emotions to work with (page 197): Forgiveness 200, Honor 202, Respect 205, Confidence 198

Colors to work with (page 211): Green 213, Yellow 221, Orange 216

## Rib Cage

### Possible Contributing Factors

Feeling stuck, overburdened, consumed by constant self-doubt that sabotages your plans. Life structures built on fear, limitation, and control.

## Remedy

Rub your hands together. When you feel your hands tingling, place them over your rib cage. Imagine that the most beautiful rays of green, healing light coming out of your right hand and a white, purifying light coming out of your left hand. Focus on your breathing. Every time you breathe in, focus on expanding your entire rib cage to allow the rays to fill it with healing, regenerative light. Each time you exhale, focus on releasing all density and tension. Embrace new possibilities.

Say: "Divine Healing Intelligence, please help me release all feelings of stuckness, fear, control, burden, limitation, self-doubt, and sabotage from my rib cage, as well as all points of view, all patterns, and the positive and negative charges that contribute to this condition." Repeat the word "CLEAR" until you feel a shift occur.

Say: "Divine Healing Intelligence, please help me discover my spontaneous, free, and flexible nature. Allow me to find new ways of thinking and seeing life, and transform all doubts into faith and self-confidence. Thank you."

Say: "Divine Healing Intelligence, please heal and regenerate my rib cage to its maximum health, vitality, and well-being."

Unhealthy emotions to work with (page 171): Stuckness 196, Low Self-Esteem 190, Fear 179, Control 174
Healthy emotions to work with (page 197): Freedom 201, Confidence 198, Clarity 197
Colors to work with (page 211): White 220, Green 213, Yellow 221

## Shins

### Possible Contributing Factors

Anger, weakness, feelings of betrayal, victimhood, and disloyalty. Carrying guilt, self-punishment, self-sacrifice. Wanting revenge, justice, fairness.

### Remedy

Say: "Divine Healing Intelligence, please release all anger, guilt, self-punishment, victimhood, and feelings of betrayal out of my shins, as well as all points of view, all patterns, and the positive and negative charges that contribute to this condition." Repeat the word "CLEAR" until you feel a shift occur.

Say: "Divine Healing Intelligence, please install feelings of inner strength, self-empowerment, and self-love. Help me bring back a sense of innocence, purity, and joy. Thank you."

Say: "Divine Healing Intelligence, please heal and regenerate my shins, legs, and ankles to their maximum health, vitality, and well-being."

*See also* Ankles, Legs.

Unhealthy emotions to work with (page 171): Guilt 184, Anger 173, Judgment 188
Healthy emotions to work with (page 197): Forgiveness 200, Honor 202, Support 206
Colors to work with (page 211): Green 213, Pink 217

## Shoulders

### Possible Contributing Factors
Carrying the weight of the world. Holding on to too much strain, stress, and worry. Feeling insecure, unsure, frightened, overwhelmed, sad, rejected, distrustful, and discouraged. Easily hurt. Droopy shoulders, indicating a lack of joy and fun. Seriousness. Focusing on problems rather than solutions.

### Remedy
Focus your attention on your shoulders. How do they feel? Are they tight or relaxed? Become aware of all the responsibility you carry on your shoulders. Close your eyes, breathe deeply, and imagine the release of all your worries, as if they were big rocks that you can throw away. Use your hands to take the rocks off of your shoulders, and throw them into an imaginary ocean.

Say: "Divine Healing Intelligence, please release all the strain, stress, worry, insecurity, confusion, hurt, rejection, and sadness from my shoulders, as well as all points of view, all patterns, and the positive and negative charges that contribute to this condition." Repeat the word "CLEAR" until you feel a shift occur.

Take a deep breath in and tighten your shoulders. Hold your breath for five seconds, then exhale slowly and completely relax your shoulders. Do this several times until they feel lighter. Next, rotate your right shoulder forward in a counterclockwise motion for fifteen seconds; rest for fifteen seconds. Repeat this three times. Now do the same rotation toward the back in a clockwise motion for the same amount of time. Repeat this process for the left shoulder.

Say: "Divine Healing Intelligence, please install courage, balance, confidence, and joy into my life. Help me find blessings and opportunities even in the most challenging experiences. Thank you."

Allow yourself to completely relax for a few minutes. Imagine that you are standing in warm, yellow sunlight. Allow the rays to penetrate deep into your shoulders, softening the muscles and dissolving all tension.

Say: "Divine Healing Intelligence, please heal and regenerate my shoulders to their full strength, vitality, and mobility."

Unhealthy emotions to work with (page 171): Stress 194, Worry 197, Fear 179, Feeling Overwhelmed 180

Healthy emotions to work with (page 197): Peace 204, Relaxation 205, Compassion 198, Support 206

Colors to work with (page 211): Green 213, Yellow 221, Blue 211

## Sinuses

### Possible Contributing Factors
Feeling irritated, frustrated with other people, in need of your own space. Difficulty standing up for yourself and saying what you believe. Feeling pulled in different directions, with too much going on, causing you to feel torn, exhausted, worn out. Thinking too much, rather than feeling or tuning in to your Divine Wisdom.

### Remedy
Say: "Divine Healing Intelligence, please release all irritation, frustration, lack of self-confidence, emotional perplexity, and exhaustion from my sinuses, as well as all

points of view, all patterns, and the positive and negative charges that contribute to this condition." Repeat the word "CLEAR" until you feel a shift occur.

In order to relieve sinus problems, colds, coughs, or asthma, place your palms together and clasp your fingers. Allow one thumb to remain upright. Encircle this thumb with the index finger and thumb of your other hand. Take slow, deep breaths. Hold this position five to fifteen minutes, several times a day.

Say: "Divine Healing Intelligence, please allow me to feel safe, protected, clear, content, and in charge of my life. Help me to value and look after myself in a loving, caring, and gentle manner. Thank you."

Say: "Divine Healing Intelligence, please clear and heal my sinuses and respiratory system to their maximum health, vitality, and well-being."

*See also* Nose.

Unhealthy emotions to work with (page 171): Stress 194, Worry 197, Fear 179, Feeling Overwhelmed 180, Low Self-Esteem 190
Healthy emotions to work with (page 197): Peace 204, Relaxation 205, Respect 205, Confidence 198
Colors to work with (page 211): Purple 217, Indigo 214, Violet 220

## Skeleton

### Possible Contributing Factors
Judgment of self and others. Feeling let down, betrayed, taken advantage of, duped. Holding on to secrets; being dishonest with yourself and others.

### Remedy
What skeletons are you keeping in the closet? What pain have you not resolved from past friendships and relationships? This is an opportunity to resolve these issues—to heal and move forward—or to degenerate further and be stuck in the past. You can do this by being completely honest with yourself, and by journaling or meditating.

Close your eyes and ask for a healing guide to assist you. When you see or sense a presence, ask your guide to take you to a healing room. When you enter the room, sit down and ask for advice and assistance with your problems. Be open to receiving healing messages, either immediately or later, through signs that will be visible to you.

Say: "Divine Healing Intelligence, I ask you to release all feelings of betrayal, dishonesty, judgments, unresolved pain, and deception from my skeleton, as well as all points of view, all patterns, and the positive and negative charges that contribute to this condition." Repeat the word "CLEAR" until you feel a shift occur.

As you let go of past pain, observe that the skeletons you have been keeping in your closet have dissolved and no longer drain your energy.

Say: "Divine Healing Intelligence, please install feelings of clarity, honesty, and support. Allow me to become more empowered and to live with integrity, honesty, and openness. Thank you."

Visualize bathing your skeleton in beautiful emerald rays of light. Observe your skeleton absorbing the healing energy of the rays to become stronger and regenerate.

Say: "Divine Healing Intelligence, please heal and regenerate my skeleton to its maximum strength, flexibility, and well-being."

Unhealthy emotions to work with (page 171): Judgment 188, Low Self-Esteem 190, Resentment 192
Healthy emotions to work with (page 197): Support 206, Recognition 204, Faith 199
Colors to work with (page 211): Green 213, Pink 217, Purple 217, Silver 219

## *Skin*

### Possible Contributing Factors
Failure to protect or be protected. Feeling irritated, angry, frustrated—like someone or something is getting under your skin. Disapproval, criticism, invalidation, or even hatred of self. Timid, withdrawn, insecure; feeling second best, devalued, uncomfortable in your own skin. Feeling like you don't belong and putting up barriers to guard yourself.

## Remedy

Who or what is getting under your skin? What are you not expressing that you need to say? To find out, stand in front of a mirror. Close your eyes and imagine that you are standing next to someone who loves you. If you could borrow their eyes, how would you see yourself? When you feel positive, open your eyes and look at yourself from the perspective of love. How do you see yourself differently? What does a person who loves you see? Affirm that you are lovable.

Now lie or sit, and close your eyes. Imagine that you hold a laser beam made of different colors in your hands. Visualize moving this light onto any area of your skin that is irritated, dry, swollen, itchy, or spotty. Observe the light changing color according to the part of the body the laser is treating. For example, if the skin is red, the laser may change to blue to counteract the redness. If the skin is dry, the laser may change to pink to regenerate the area; or if the skin is swollen, orange rays are great to calm the swelling. And if the skin is itchy, yellow rays can help to soothe it. Focus on letting go of all anger, frustration, self-criticism, irritation, and dislike of yourself.

Say: "Divine Healing Intelligence, please release all irritation, anger, frustration, criticism, invalidation, and insecurity I carry in my skin, as well as all points of view, all patterns, and the positive and negative charges that contribute to this condition." Repeat the word "CLEAR" until you feel a shift occur.

In your mind's eye, observe your skin beginning to clear, becoming radiant, lustrous, glowing, and soft. How does it feel to have this new skin? Allow yourself to take long deep breaths and to enjoy your renewed skin.

Say: "Divine Healing Intelligence, please allow me to feel comfortable, happy, and secure in my skin. Allow me to learn to love, appreciate, and value myself. Thank you."

Focus on feeling comfortable and secure with your new skin.

To improve your skin's texture, touch the tip of your ring finger with the tip of your thumb. Straighten the other fingers. Hold this position for two to three minutes while taking slow, deep breaths. Do it two to three times a day.

Say: "Divine Healing Intelligence, please remove all toxicity, bacteria, impurities, and stress from my skin, and regenerate my skin and all related organs to their maximum health, vitality, and well-being."

Even if you don't see instant results, keep doing this exercise to allow yourself to become comfortable with who you are. You will see changes in both your skin and your self-confidence.

Unhealthy emotions to work with (page 171): Stress 194, Worry 197, Fear 179, Feeling Overwhelmed 180

Healthy emotions to work with (page 197): Peace 204, Satisfaction 206, Confidence 198, Happiness 201

Colors to work with (page 211): Yellow 221, Blue 211, White 220, Indigo 214, Purple 217, Turquoise 219

## Small Intestine

### Possible Contributing Factors

Feeling abandoned, insecure, easily distracted, vulnerable, confused, bloated. Participating in relentless self-sabotage and procrastination. Feeling scattered, stuck, lost. Pining for unrequited love.

### Remedy

Say: "Divine Healing Intelligence, I ask you to release all feelings of insecurity, abandonment, and confusion. Please help me to let go of all self-sabotage, distraction, stuckness, and procrastination from my small intestine as well as all points of view, all patterns, and the positive and negative charges that contribute to this condition." Repeat the word "CLEAR" until you feel a shift occur.

Say: "Divine Healing Intelligence, please install feelings of security, lightness, well-being, and focus. Help me to become clear, determined, and centered. Allow me to love and appreciate myself, and the people around me. Thank you."

Say: "Divine Healing Intelligence, please heal and regenerate my small intestine to its maximum health, vitality, and well-being."

*See also* Bowels.

Unhealthy emotions to work with (page 171): Stuckness 196, Low Self-Esteem 190, Fear 179

Healthy emotions to work with (page 197): Clarity 197, Freedom 201, Confidence 198

Colors to work with (page 211): Orange 216, Green 213, Brown 212, Yellow 221

## Spine

### Possible Contributing Factors

Feeling weak, confused, fearful, and insecure. Difficulty communicating with others and asking for what you want. Feeling unsupported and alone. Not knowing who or where to ask for help. Feeling that the world is an unsafe place to live in. Trying to protect yourself from pain and hurt. Feeling stuck in a pattern or situation you can't get out of.

### Cervical Spine—Neck Region

**C1**—Feelings of fear, confusion, fight-or-flight; wanting to run away from problems and responsibilities. Feeling insecure, not good enough, too focused on other people's opinions. Taking on other people's problems, difficulty saying no, playing mind games. On the physical level: headaches, migraines, difficulty sleeping, dizziness, exhaustion, nervous breakdowns, or anxiety attacks due to the effect of negative feelings on the sympathetic nervous system, pituitary gland, brain, and middle ear.

**C2**—Feeling rejected, inflexible; thinking that you know better than others. Can't make up your mind; feel frustrated, angry, resentful. Trying to find a scapegoat. Feeling unbalanced, discouraged, depressed, disempowered, disconnected with your spiritual energy. On the physical level: allergies, earaches, deafness, fainting, as well as problems with eyes or sinuses.

**C3**—Buying into other people's negative beliefs. Judging yourself and others. Feeling insecure, vulnerable, indecisive. Experiencing low self-esteem; feeling limited, impatient, irritated. Propensity to grind your teeth. On the physical level: ear, teeth, jaw, headache, or skin issues such as acne, pimples, eczema. An example of an ear problem may be a fullness in the ear, decreased hearing, tinnitus, and vertigo.

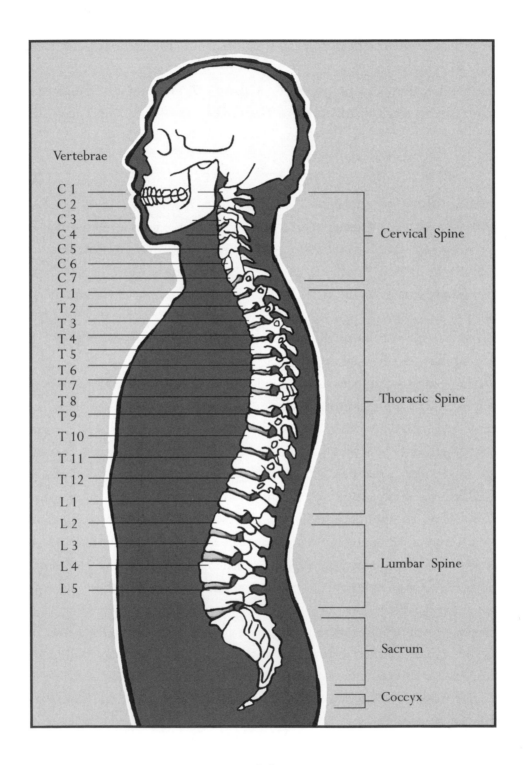

Vertebrae

C 1
C 2
C 3
C 4
C 5
C 6
C 7
T 1
T 2
T 3
T 4
T 5
T 6
T 7
T 8
T 9
T 10
T 11
T 12
L 1
L 2
L 3
L 4
L 5

Cervical Spine

Thoracic Spine

Lumbar Spine

Sacrum

Coccyx

**C4**—Thinking that life isn't fair; carrying old guilt, unresolved pain, and sadness, especially with those close to you. Stressing too much and feeling overwhelmed. Suppressing your feelings of anger, and then erupting. On the physical level: hay fever, catarrh, adenoids, deafness, mouth ulcers, sinusitis.

**C5**—Fear of being wrong. Dreading humiliation, embarrassment, or ridicule. Difficulty expressing yourself because of your great concern about what others may think. Regular self-sabotage, low self-worth, difficulty accepting good things into your life. Feeling overburdened, strained, and limited. On the physical level: vocal cord problems, laryngitis, hoarseness, a sore throat.

**C6**—Feeling overwhelmed by worries, anxieties, and stresses. Rather than dealing with your own issues, meddling in other people's lives to fix their problems and take attention away from yours. Resisting life, feeling stuck, afraid to let go of old fears and change. On the physical level: a stiff neck, shoulder pain, tonsillitis, whooping cough.

**C7**—Feeling tired, uninspired, drained, emotionally wound up, mentally unclear. Immobilized by negativity, lack, and fear of the future. Feeling numb and disconnected from your own truth and sense of power. On the physical level: thyroid problems, colds, shoulder pain, frozen shoulder, elbow issues.

## Thoracic Spine—Mid-Back Region

**T1**—Feeling overwhelmed by responsibilities; wanting to run and hide, and let someone else take over. Difficulty letting go and trusting. Inability to find your center. On the physical level: pain in your arms, hands, wrists, and fingers; colds, difficulty breathing, shortness of breath; and, in acute cases, asthma that develops over time.

**T2**—Feeling shut down, and unable to fully give and receive love. Controlling, protecting the heart from hurt, holding on to pain and heartbreak from the past. Distrusting, always on guard, thinking that someone is working against you and is going to hurt you. Inability to love or nurture yourself. Holding on to too much fear and worry; feeling helpless and hopeless, like a victim of your life. On the physical level: chest infections as well as heart problems, including complications with the arteries and valves.

**T3**—Feeling confused, scared, scattered, and lost. Difficulty finding the right words to express yourself. Suppressing old sadness and anger. Acting the slave to others while letting them take advantage of you. Always putting yourself last, which leads to exhaustion and burnout. Relying too much on the opinions of others, instead of learning to trust and value your own wisdom, inner guidance, and intuition. On the physical level: chest congestion, influenza, and upper and lower respiratory infections.

**T4**—Feeling irritated, annoyed, and frustrated that your life is full of struggle and seemingly insurmountable challenges. May be experiencing feelings of jealousy toward others and envy at how easy their lives seem compared with yours. Judging yourself and others harshly, looking at the negative side of life. Carrying unresolved pain and trauma from the past. Afraid to heal or let go, as this life is all you know. On the physical level: gallbladder problems, jaundice, shingles.

**T5**—Feeling stuck, like things are not moving in the right direction. Giving too much focus to the outside world and what it has to offer you. In need of time to become aware of your emotions and work through them, rather than simply stuffing them down because they're too hard to deal with. Too much pressure and stress on your body and emotional well-being due to lack of attention. On the physical level: liver problems, fevers, low blood pressure, poor circulation, arthritis, and food addictions.

**T6**—Carrying too many burdens, stresses, and problems. Stuck in the belief system that loving someone means worrying about them constantly. Feeling overpowered and controlled by others. Believing that you have to stay in a situation because there is no choice. Fearful of disappointment, failure, or rejection. Thinking that others know better than you but secretly wanting to prove them wrong. Difficulty making empowering decisions. On the physical level: stomach problems, indigestion, heartburn, bloating, feelings of heaviness, and weight problems/obesity.

**T7**—Carrying bitterness, resentment, and feelings of victimhood. Feeling unworthy of having great things in your life. Impatiently searching for a quick fix and then feeling disappointed when it doesn't work. Feeling like you have to prove yourself to others in order to gain their acceptance. Overcautious, taking life too seriously. Needing to inject more humor and fun into your days. On the physical level: pancreas and duodenum problems, diabetes, ulcers, or gastritis.

**T8**—Unsatisfied with life but resistant to change. Too easily influenced by other people, although extremely stubborn and unyielding once your mind is made up. Very sensitive and easily hurt, often misinterpreting what others say. Afraid of failure and of looking stupid in front of people. Holding grudges and then looking for someone to blame. On the physical level: spleen and immune system problems, mucus congestion, a cough, lack of energy and vitality.

**T9**—Not honoring yourself and your needs. Doing rather than being. Trying to impress others by overextending yourself and then feeling burned out. Looking for approval. Feeling out of sync with life. Alternating between feeling overexcited to depressed, hopeful to hopeless, happy to sad. Perfectionism. On the physical level: problems with adrenal glands, fatigue, allergies, hives.

**T10**—Living in the past and holding on to feelings of resentment, anger, judgment, and blame. Feeling that if you hold on to your anger, it will hurt the other person, rather than seeing how it hurts you and keeps you stuck. Refusal to change and see the other person's point of view. Selfishness, arrogance, and righteousness. On the physical level: kidney problems, chronic tiredness, hardening of the arteries.

**T11**—Low self-esteem, difficulty fitting in and feeling accepted. Afraid that people will take advantage of you and hurt you. Feeling second best, like something is wrong with you. Difficulty communicating your needs in relationships. Often attracting abusive relationships. On the physical level: kidney problems, acne, pimples, eczema.

**T12**—Feeling insecure, fearful, lost. Difficulty digesting life. Often sabotaging yourself and your possible successes. Deep-seated belief that you deserve to suffer and struggle. Holding on to guilt from the past, which stops you from moving forward. On the physical level: problems with the small intestine, rheumatism, infertility.

*Lumbar Spine—Lower Back Region*

**L1**—Feeling poisoned by resentment, stagnation, and unresolved issues from the past. Thoughts and words don't align with your actions, leading to feelings of confusion, depression, criticism, and sadness. Needing to forgive, move forward, and take positive action in order to heal. On the physical level: constipation, colitis, diarrhea, hernias.

**L2**—Feeling like there is little or no choice, a sense of giving up. Too much focus on the outside world and what you're not getting, rather than on your inner strength.

Needing to deal with your childhood pain and low self-esteem. Feeling powerless in your situation and pushing yourself over your limit. On the physical level: abdominal and upper leg pain, appendicitis, cramps, difficulty breathing, varicose veins.

**L3**—Feeling either lack of desire or too much desire with no outlet. Trying to sweep unresolved issues under the carpet and pretend they don't matter, rather than dealing with them. Disconnecting from your emotions so that you don't feel the rejection, fear, anger, and frustration you are suppressing. Tendency to erupt in angry and judgmental outbursts. Extremely sensitive about what others say about you. Rejection of the feminine energy for females and masculine energy for males. Problems with communication and commitment in relationships. Experiencing chaos, lack of clarity, and resistance. Caught up in your point of view. On the physical level: bladder problems, incontinence, knee pain, sexual dysfunction, and problems with the reproductive system, such as painful periods and impotency.

**L4**—A sense of disempowerment with work and family. Pressure to have enough money and to provide for others. Struggling with finances. Feeling overwhelmed and confused as to what action to take. Difficulty valuing yourself. Allowing others to dictate your worth. Finding too many excuses for why things should stay as they are. Difficulty completing projects. Fear of failure. Either abstaining from or obsessed by sex. On the physical level: prostate problems, lower back pain, sciatica, difficulty/pain during urination.

**L5**—Feeling weak, confused, weighed down—as if something is holding you back and you are unable to move forward. Holding on to feelings of betrayal, abandonment, and isolation. Difficulty trusting people and following through with your plans. Frequent self-sabotage, anger, and anxiety. A tendency to see yourself as a victim. On the physical level: problems with your legs, poor circulation, swollen or weak ankles, cold feet, leg cramps.

*Sacrum*
Feeling unsupported, carrying unresolved family issues, holding on to childhood anger and resentment. Experiencing a lack of confidence and belief in self. Feeling uncom-

fortable in your body and in your life. Carrying guilt, resentment, and shame. On the physical level: problems with hips and buttocks, spinal curvature.

### Coccyx

Feeling unbalanced; focused on how life is unfair and you can't get what you want. Blaming others and life circumstances for your challenges, mistakes, and failures. Easily depressed, disappointed, and disillusioned. Feeling betrayed or cheated. Frequently sabotaging yourself, and plunging into negativity and fear. Life seems monotonous and repetitive; nothing much seems to change. Loss of direction and self-confidence. On the physical level: problems with the rectum or anus, such as hemorrhoids.

### Remedy

Touch any sore point on your spine, take a deep breath in, and visualize any stuckness releasing. Then massage lengthwise along the side of your feet, from the big toe to the heel, as this part of your feet relates to your spine. Continue to focus on the parts that are sore. When you are massaging a sore point, close your eyes, take in a few deep breaths, and focus on the color green. Visualize the green dissolving the blockage, which may appear dark in color. Then focus on the sore point in your spine, breathe into it, and flood it with green light.

Say: "Divine Healing Intelligence, please dissolve all pain, stress, and tension from my spine (if you want to be specific, ask that it be released from the part of your spine which is hurting, such as L2). I ask that all the vertebrae in my spine now come into alignment." Repeat the word "CLEAR" until you feel a shift occur.

*See also* Back.

Unhealthy emotions to work with (page 171): Work with emotions related to the vertebrae you are focusing on

Healthy emotions to work with (page 197): Confidence 198, Relaxation 205, Recognition 204, Support 206, Satisfaction 206, and others which relate to the vertebrae you are focusing on

Colors to work with (page 211): Green 213, Yellow 221, Blue 211

## *Spleen*

### Possible Contributing Factors

Feeling helpless, disconnected from feminine energy, fearful, frozen, angry, frustrated. Overly sensitive and easily swayed. Constantly trying to find fault in others, and control or change them. Not wanting to face your own issues and participate in life fully. Continually worrying and stressing about others.

### Remedy

Close your eyes and make a fist with both hands. Place your thumbs over your ring fingers. Focus on the feelings of anger, frustration, helplessness, and fear that are stuck in your spleen and in your body. Breathe deeply as you allow yourself to fully connect with these feelings. Do this for thirty to sixty seconds. Tighten your whole body for ten to twenty seconds, then completely relax and open your palms. Repeat this process several times until you feel more relaxed.

Say: "Divine Healing Intelligence, I ask you to release all helplessness, fear, frustration, control, and dissatisfaction from my spleen, as well as all points of view, all patterns, and the positive and negative charges that contribute to this condition." Repeat the word "CLEAR" until you feel a shift occur.

Focus on receiving from the universe all the help, strength, confidence, and satisfaction you desire. Allow it to flow into your hands. Visualize colors coming into your hands and attributes that you need to become happier, to achieve health, and to attract the finances or other resources you require. Allow yourself to be showered with the energy of abundance and possibility.

Place your hands on your spleen. Massage it for a few minutes while repeating, "Heal, clear, regenerate now."

Say: "Divine Healing Intelligence, please help me to listen to my wisdom, and to make healing, empowering, and excellent decisions which will allow me to experience a more fulfilling life. Thank you."

Say: "Divine Healing Intelligence, please heal and regenerate my spleen and all related organs to their maximum health, vitality, and well-being."

## *Stomach*

### Possible Contributing Factors

Difficulty digesting life and assimilating new information. Feeling stuck in a pattern of fear, limitation, worry, guilt, and despair. Behaving in a superior, arrogant, controlling way; thinking that you are better than others; or feeling inferior and second best. At times self-obsessed and demanding, wanting everything your own way. Difficulty expressing yourself and dealing with rejection. Feeling attacked, like you've been punched in the stomach.

### Remedy

Place your attention on your stomach; become aware of how it feels. If your stomach had a voice and could tell you how it felt, what would it say? What feelings, energies or experiences are you holding in your stomach that cause you pain? Imagine there is a purple fire in front of you. Visualize taking all the worry, nervousness, attack, guilt, stuckness, rejection, and pain from your stomach and putting it into this purple fire.

Say: "Divine Healing Intelligence, I ask you to release all despair, nervousness, worry, arrogance, guilt, rejection, and attack from my stomach, as well as all points of view, all patterns, and the positive and negative charges that contribute to this condition." Repeat the word "CLEAR" until you feel a shift occur.

Slowly massage the index finger of your right hand from base to tip and visualize the release of all the negativity that is stored there, throwing it into the fire. Do this for a few minutes.

Repeat several times: "I let go of all control, worry, and guilt. I welcome joy, peace, and well-being."

Visualize beautiful yellow sunlight pouring into your stomach, pacifying, clearing, and relaxing it.

Say: "Divine Healing Intelligence, please increase my faith, self-confidence, and ability to trust that life will bring me the best, most empowering, and brilliant experiences for me to learn and grow. Thank you."

To help ease digestive problems, simply massage the tip of your nose with your middle finger in a circular fashion, putting as much pressure as you feel comfortable with. Do this for forty-five seconds, then rest for twenty-five seconds. Repeat this three to four times.

Say: "Divine Healing Intelligence, please heal and regenerate my stomach and all related organs to their maximum health, vitality, and well-being."

Unhealthy emotions to work with (page 171): Stuckness 196, Control 174, Rejection 191, Guilt 184, Attack 174

Healthy emotions to work with (page 197): Forgiveness 200, Love 203, Joy 203, Happiness 201, Encouragement 199

Colors to work with (page 211): Green 213, Yellow 221, Blue 211

## Teeth

### Possible Contributing Factors

Holding on to shame, guilt, fear, anger, blame, bitterness. Difficulty making empowering decisions. Self-neglect. Unresolved childhood issues and frequent self-sabotage. Feeling overwhelmed and stressed. Frustrated about your inability to express yourself clearly.

### Remedy

Focus on your teeth; close your eyes. Imagine that you have a small vacuum cleaner, which is able to suck out all density or toxins from your teeth. Observe as dense, heavy energy comes out of your teeth.

Say: "Divine Healing Intelligence, I ask you to release all shame, guilt, fear, neglect, blame, anger, and bitterness from my teeth, as well as all points of view, all patterns, and the positive and negative charges that contribute to this condition." Repeat the word "CLEAR" until you feel a shift occur.

If you have a toothache, touch the tip of your thumb with the tip of your little finger, and then straighten your other fingers. Do this with both hands for ten to fifteen minutes until you feel relief.

Visualize a beautiful, pearl-colored substance being placed into each tooth. This substance begins to regenerate the teeth, making them stronger and healthier.

Say: "Divine Healing Intelligence, please help me to listen to my own wisdom to make healing, empowering, and excellent decisions that allow me to experience a more fulfilling life. Thank you."

Say: "Divine Healing Intelligence, please heal and regenerate my teeth and gums to their maximum health, vitality, and well-being."

Unhealthy emotions to work with (page 171): Shame 193, Guilt 184, Fear 179, Anger 173
Healthy emotions to work with (page 197): Innocence 202, Forgiveness 200, Peace 204, Freedom 201
Colors to work with (page 211): White 220, Blue 211

## Testicles

### Possible Contributing Factors
Feeling threatened, exposed, and insecure. Unable to handle the situations life throws at you. Uncomfortable with your sexuality. Holding on to guilt, shame, anger. Difficulty forgiving and moving on.

### Remedy
With whom are you angry? What would it take for you to let go of the anger? What steps do you need to take to move forward in your life? If you are ready to let go of the pain and anger, do the forgiveness process, even if it is just to forgive yourself.

Say: "Divine Healing Intelligence, I ask you to release all feelings of negativity, insecurity, guilt, anger, threat, and shame which are stored in my testicles, as well as all points of view, all patterns, and the positive and negative charges that contribute to this condition." Repeat the word "CLEAR" until you feel a shift occur.

Stand, keeping your spine straight. Rub your hands together, then hold them slightly apart. Visualize green light coming out of your palms. Place your hands palms down, with your fingers close together and your middle fingers just touching your testicles. Take slow, deep breaths as you concentrate on energizing and regenerating your testicles with the green light. Do this for three to five minutes.

Say: "Divine Healing Intelligence, please help me feel comfortable with my sexuality, and masculinity. Allow me to move through life with ease, grace, and confidence. Thank you."

Say: "Divine Healing Intelligence, please heal and regenerate my testicles to their maximum health, vitality, and well-being."

Unhealthy emotions to work with (page 171): Shame 193, Guilt 184, Fear 179, Anger 173

Healthy emotions to work with (page 197): Forgiveness 200, Honor 202, Peace 204, Freedom 201

Colors to work with (page 211): Green 213, Orange 216, Yellow 221

## Thalamus

### Possible Contributing Factors

Feeling disconnected from your authentic self. Difficulty communicating with or understanding others. Feeling like everything is piling on top of you. Feeling messy, chaotic, confused. Feeling that your work lacks recognition. Invalidating, dishonoring, disempowering yourself. Difficulty making clear choices.

### Remedy

Say: "Divine Healing Intelligence, I ask you to release all feelings of disconnection, chaos, invalidation, confusion, and limitation from my thalamus, as well as all points of view, all patterns, and the positive and negative charges that contribute to this condition." Repeat the word "CLEAR" until you feel a shift occur.

Sit up. Interlock your fingers and move your thumbs away from your index fingers. Raise your hands above your head, with your thumbs facing the back of your head. Extend your thumbs toward the back of your head. Hold the posture for one to two minutes. Visualize a bright yellow light moving from your hands into your thalamus. Take slow, deep breaths. Allow the light to regenerate your thalamus and bring it into perfect working order.

Say: "Divine Healing Intelligence, please install feelings of clarity, connection, and well-being, and a sense of organization and recognition. Thank you."

Say: "Divine Healing Intelligence, please heal and regenerate my thalamus and all related organs to their maximum health, vitality, and well-being."

*See also* Brain.

Unhealthy emotions to work with (page 171): Stuckness 196, Stress 194, Worry 197
Healthy emotions to work with (page 197): Clarity 197, Relaxation 205, Peace 204
Colors to work with (page 211): Indigo 214, White 220, Purple 217, Yellow 221

## *Thighs*

### Possible Contributing Factors
Inability to give birth to new ideas. Overcritical, negative, judgmental, and limited in your point of view. Feeling suppressed, rejected, stuck, fearful, neglectful. Difficulty nurturing and taking care of yourself.

### Remedy
Focus on your thighs; gently massage them. As you do, become aware of all the harmful judgment and criticism you carry about your thighs. Each time you have a negative thought, imagine that it is a weed that needs to be pulled. Picture yourself ripping out these weeds.

Say: "Divine Healing Intelligence, I ask you to release all criticism, negativity, judgment, lack, stuckness, and fear from my thighs, as well as all points of view, all patterns, and the positive and negative charges that contribute to this condition." Repeat the word "CLEAR" until you feel a shift occur.

Now, focus on enjoying your body. Tell your thighs how much you appreciate them. Thank them for the wonderful job they do supporting and carrying you.

Say: "Divine Healing Intelligence, please help me give birth to new, wonderful, creative ideas. Allow me to become more positive and joyful, and more willing to participate in life's adventures. Thank you."

Massage your thighs. Visualize a strong, silver light moving through them to provide strength and regeneration.

Say: "Divine Healing Intelligence, please heal and regenerate my thighs to their maximum health, vitality, and well-being."

Unhealthy emotions to work with (page 171): Rejection 191, Stuckness 196, Fear 179, Judgment 188

Healthy emotions to work with (page 197): Faith 199, Freedom 201, Support 206, Happiness 201

Colors to work with (page 211): Orange 216, Green 213, Silver 219

## Throat

### Possible Contributing Factors

Difficulty communicating, low self-esteem, self-doubt, self-sabotage. Feeling shut down, misunderstood, held back, fearful, frustrated, stuck, unworthy of good things. In conflict with self and continually changing your mind. Difficulty trusting. Feeling depressed, sad, hopeless, uncreative, and uninspired. Thinking that you lack choice.

### Remedy

Place your attention on your throat. Breathe in to it. Now, imagine there is a fire that surrounds the back of your throat. Bring your focus to the fire, and place all pain, soreness, fear, low self-esteem, distrust, judgments, and lack into the red fire. Allow them to burn.

Say: "Divine Healing Intelligence, please assist me to release all feelings of unworthiness, sadness, self-doubt, and lack of choice from my throat, as well as all points of view, all patterns, and the positive and negative charges that contribute to this condition." Repeat the word "CLEAR" until you feel a shift occur.

Now, imagine that there is a big blue bubble that surrounds the front of your throat. Focus on that bubble. Allow it to surround your throat like a soft blue cloud. Let the softness of the cloud float into your throat, filling it with confidence and the ability to speak strongly, honestly, lovingly, clearly, and expressively.

Say: "Divine Healing Intelligence, please strengthen and improve my communication abilities. Help me open up to wonderful new possibilities, enhanced relationships, and greater self-confidence. Thank you."

Observe the cloud transforming into a loudspeaker in front of your throat so that everything you say can be heard by others. You must be willing to communicate an empowering message from your heart to ensure that what you communicate will benefit others and yourself.

If you have a sore throat, you may want to try a lion posture from yoga to help you heal quickly. Kneel and sit back on your heels, pressing your palms firmly on your knees and spreading your fingers as far apart as you can. Inhale deeply through your nose, open your mouth wide, and stick your tongue out, curling it toward your chin. Open your eyes wide and stiffen your fingers. Exhale slowly through your mouth while making a roaring "HA!" sound. Repeat this posture five or six times.

Say: "Divine Healing Intelligence, please heal and regenerate my throat to its maximum health, vitality, and well-being."

Unhealthy emotions to work with (page 171): Stress 194, Worry 197, Fear 179, Feeling Overwhelmed 180

Healthy emotions to work with (page 197): Encouragement 199, Confidence 198, Clarity 197

Colors to work with (page 211): Turquoise 219, Blue 211, Orange 216

## *Thymus Gland*

### Possible Contributing Factors
Buying into lies and false ideas. Lacking integrity. Accumulation of nervous stress, tension, and worry. Difficulty taking responsibility for your actions. Playing the victim. Feeling unhappy, low, vulnerable, tired, and emotionally up and down.

### Remedy
Close your eyes and tune into your thymus gland. Become aware of any density or heaviness stored there. Using the orange flame of light, visualize dissolving all density and tension from your thymus.

Say: "Divine Healing Intelligence, I ask you to release all feelings of nervousness, unhappiness, instability, lies, worries, and stress from my thymus gland, as well as all points of view, all patterns, and the positive and negative charges that contribute to this condition." Repeat the word "CLEAR" until you feel a shift occur.

To improve your thymus gland, concentrate on it and smile. The more you smile and the happier you are, the better your thymus will work. Now, think of something that makes you laugh or feel really happy, and smile again. To help stimulate your thymus further, place two fingers on top of the thymus and tap fifteen to twenty times while still smiling.

Say: "Divine Healing Intelligence, please strengthen my immune system and over-all health. Allow me to transform nervousness into calm, instability into stability, and lies into truth. Thank you."

Say: "Divine Healing Intelligence, please heal and regenerate my thymus and all related glands to their maximum health, vitality, and well-being."

Unhealthy emotions to work with (page 171): Stuckness 196, Stress 194, Worry 197, Anxiety 174, Criticism 175

Healthy emotions to work with (page 197): Relaxation 205, Clarity 197, Peace 204, Freedom 201

Colors to work with (page 211): Orange 216, Green 213, Pink 217

## Thyroid Gland

### Possible Contributing Factors

Lack of drive; feeling sluggish, numb, disconnected from your life's purpose. Holding back, and constantly trying to please others by carrying their burdens and worries. Muddled thinking. Feeling emotionally unstable, up and down, and confused. Constantly playing a game of guilt and punishment. Sabotaging yourself. Wasting a lot of time doing things in an inefficient manner, which drains your energy. Never enough time to get everything done.

### Remedy

Focus on your thyroid. What are you holding back and not expressing? Whose worries or burdens are you carrying in your thyroid? What do you want to do that you are not doing?

Become aware of any blockages; you may visualize these as ropes or chains around your thyroid. Imagine that a huge fire is in front of you. Take all the chains and ropes off your thyroid and throw them into the fire. Make sure you also dissolve all your burdens, worries, and stresses about other people.

Say: "Divine Healing Intelligence, I ask you to release all feelings of numbness, lack of drive, tiredness, instability, and confusion from my thyroid, as well as all points of view, all patterns, and the positive and negative charges that contribute to this condition." Repeat the word "CLEAR" until you feel a shift occur.

Visualize beautiful indigo light as a soft scarf surrounding your thyroid and repairing it. Allow the indigo to awaken your energy, vitality, and thirst for life.

Place your index fingers on your thyroid glands, which are situated on either side of the windpipe, near your collarbone. Massage your thyroid glands in a circular motion, moving up and down the throat. Do this for one to two minutes.

Say: "Divine Healing Intelligence, I welcome vitality, balance, courage, and peace into my life. Thank you."

Say: "Divine Healing Intelligence, please heal and regenerate my thyroid and all related glands to their maximum health, vitality, and well-being."

## Toes

### Possible Contributing Factors

Judgment, rejection, feelings of not belonging. Feeling lost and unsure of yourself; wanting to curl up and hide. Holding too much stress and tension.

### Right Foot

**Big toe**—Confused direction in life. Asking yourself, *Where am I going?* Feeling stuck, fearful of moving forward; dragging outdated beliefs about life, money, and security from the past. Inability to express yourself clearly. On the physical level: problems with the throat, thyroid, neck, jaw, teeth, gums, and tongue.

**Second toe**—Worries, and feelings of inferiority and insecurity. Difficulty belonging to a group or to a cause. Judging yourself and others; watching your step; feeling second best, not knowing who to trust or who to listen to. On the physical level: problems with the lungs, heart, breasts, thymus gland, and shoulders.

**Third toe**—Experiencing a lack of clarity about a situation; difficulty seeing the future, especially in relation to your work or financial situation. Unrealistic expectations, feeling like a failure, or struggling to step forward. On the physical level: problems with the liver, gallbladder, pancreas, and stomach.

**Fourth toe**—Feelings of tiredness, confusion, anxiety, and depression—like a small child who wants to hide from life. Too many events and situations over which you have no control. Wanting to give up and run away, except there is nowhere to run. On the physical level: problems with digestion, and the bladder and spleen; lower back pain.

**Little toe**—Suppressed aggression. Belief that life is a struggle and that you have to work hard. Feeling unworthy of the good things in life, neglected, and abandoned.

Lacking self-worth. On the physical level: issues with the nervous system, urinary tract, rectum, circulatory system, skin, or reproductive system, such as headaches, chronic lower back pain, sciatica, depression, or sexual dysfunction.

### Left Foot

**Big toe**—Feeling overwhelmed and confused about choices made, as if there is a blurry line between what you think is right and wrong. Feeling too much responsibility; holding on to tension, stress, and worry. Not knowing who to turn to and how to express yourself. On the physical level: problems with the throat, thyroid, mouth, esophagus, jaw, ears, tongue, teeth, and gums.

**Second toe**—Confused about people and their motivations. Uncertain of the direction you need to move in. Afraid to initiate change. Difficulty with intimacy. Holding unresolved grief and heartbreak. Continual self-sabotage. On the physical level: problems with the heart, lungs, breasts, arms, shoulders, and thymus.

**Third toe**—Feeling suppression, shame, anger, low self-worth, limitation, and lack of choices. Focusing too much on past regrets and what you could have done differently. Holding back forgiveness, sweeping problems under the carpet, creating an inability to expand and move forward. Thinking and analyzing too much with inadequate action. On the physical level: problems with the stomach, liver, pancreas, gallbladder, and spleen.

**Fourth toe**—Feeling out of control and misunderstood. Holding on to victim consciousness—a "Why is this happening to me?" attitude. Can't see a way out of a situation. Belief that there is something wrong with you. Feeling rejection, guilt, lack of boundaries. On the physical level: problems with the lower back, spleen, intestines, and reproductive system.

**Little toe**—Feeling unappreciated and neglected. Self-criticizing. Feeling like a child who cannot please his or her angry parent. Belief that you can never do anything right. Feeling fearful, threatened, betrayed. Thinking, *What's the point? I might as well give up.* On the physical level: problems with the anus, bowels, large intestine, legs, immune system, and lower back.

### Remedy

To release negative or dense energies from each toe, first close your eyes and imagine that there is a fire in front of you. Using your fingers, gently pull any dense issues out of the toe you are focusing on and place the negativity (which may look like gray smoke, chains, or weeds) into the flame. You may then use the colors related to that toe to help regenerate the flow of energy.

In order to install and make the positives stronger, gently massage or hold each toe with the intention of increasing that feeling. Then, in your mind's eye, bathe the toe in the color that relates to it. Allow yourself to really feel the positive emotion you are installing.

- Big toe (throat chakra)—blue

- Second toe (heart chakra)—green

- Third toe (solar plexus chakra)—yellow

- Fourth toe (sacral chakra)—orange

- Little toe (root chakra)—red

Say: "Divine Healing Intelligence, please heal and regenerate my toes to their maximum health, vitality, and mobility."

Unhealthy emotions to work with (page 171): Any unhealthy emotion that relates to the toe you are working on

Healthy emotions to work with (page 197): Any healthy emotion that relates to the toe you are working on

Colors to work with (page 211): The colors related to the chakras or the color that you feel is most appropriate at the time

## Tongue

### Possible Contributing Factors

Not saying things you want to say because you are afraid of being judged; gossiping too much or criticizing others. Feeling uncomfortable with what you think, know, or feel. Trying to deceive yourself by pretending that everything is OK when, in actuality, changes need to be made. Feeling suppressed, abandoned, or ostracized. Difficulty speaking and standing up for yourself and your beliefs.

## Remedy

Open your mouth, stick out your tongue, and move it slowly around your lips in a circle. Repeat this five times in a clockwise motion and five times in the other direction. Focus on the tingling sensation in your tongue. For your tongue to heal and work well, it needs to be flexible.

Become aware of what you would like to say that you are not saying and to whom you would like to say it. Write this down. Now, read it out loud. Become aware of how your tongue feels as you speak these words.

Say: "Divine Healing Intelligence, please help me to dissolve all feelings of fear, judgment, abandonment, criticism, and suppression from my tongue, as well as all points of view, all patterns, and the positive and negative charges that contribute to this condition. Repeat the word "CLEAR" until you feel a shift occur.

In order to regenerate your tongue and tone your whole system, stick out your tongue and cover it with a face towel or a handkerchief. Gently pull your tongue with your hand, rotating it to the right and to the left, and then up and down. Spend forty-five seconds to a minute performing this exercise.

Say: "Divine Healing Intelligence, please help me find my voice. Allow me to speak up for what I believe in, and bring people to me who will respect me and my ideas. Thank you."

During the day, become aware of the position of your tongue and focus on relaxing it. How does that feel? Can you be angry or upset if your tongue is completely relaxed?

Say: "Divine Healing Intelligence, please heal and regenerate my tongue to its maximum flexibility, vitality, and well-being."

Unhealthy emotions to work with (page 171): Stress 194, Criticism 175, Judgment 188
Healthy emotions to work with (page 197): Flexibility and Movement 200,
    Forgiveness 200, Peace 204
Colors to work with (page 211): Orange 216, Red 218, White 220

## *Tonsils*

### Possible Contributing Factors

Needing to please others in order to be liked. Feeling like others are angry or judging you but trying to appease them by going out of your way for them. Blocking the flow of your expression and creativity. Fearing the consequences of expressing your feelings.

### Remedy

Say: "Divine Healing Intelligence, please help me to release fear, my need to please, my difficulty in expressing myself, and blocks to my creativity from my tonsils, as well as all points of view, all patterns, and the positive and negative charges that contribute to this condition." Repeat the word "CLEAR" until you feel a shift occur.

Say: "Divine Healing Intelligence, please install feelings of confidence, creativity, self-expression, and self-love. Thank you."

Say: "Divine Healing Intelligence, please heal and regenerate my tonsils to their maximum health, vitality, and well-being."

*See also* Throat.

Unhealthy emotions to work with (page 171): Anger 173, Critism 175, Judgment 188
Healthy emotions to work with (page 197): Forgiveness 200, Clarity 197, Confidence 198
Colors to work with (page 211): Orange 216, Blue 211

## *Uterus*

### Possible Contributing Factors

Discounting the feminine aspect of self, holding on to old hurts and rejection, mother issues. Feeling depleted, ungrounded, unsupported, neglected, and unbalanced. Over-concerned with other people's problems. Lack of appreciation and nurturing for self. Constant need for approval.

## Remedy

What actions can you take to begin appreciating yourself? What decisions do you need to make for your life to become happier and more balanced?

Close your eyes and tune into your uterus. If you could see it, would it look healthy and clear? If it is dense and unhealthy, imagine vacuuming all the density, disease, and disorder out.

Say: "Divine Healing Intelligence, please help me dissolve old hurts, rejection, feelings of inequality and disapproval from my uterus, as well as all points of view, all patterns, and the positive and negative charges that contribute to this condition." Repeat the word "CLEAR" until you feel a shift occur.

Imagine placing a healthy orange ball of light into your uterus. Observe it spin and clear any remaining density, regenerating and healing your uterus.

If you would like to have children, place your hands on your uterus and ask that your uterus create the best possible environment for a child. Send the energy of softness and love to your uterus. Visualize a baby growing inside you, feeling happy and joyous.

If you are unable to have children, place your hands on your abdomen. Focus on breathing into that area. Tell your reproductive system that you forgive it for not supporting your dream. Then visualize a soft yellow light surrounding your uterus and allowing it to heal.

Say: "Divine Healing Intelligence, please help me become a more dynamic, energetic, and balanced person. Help me to love and honor myself and my femininity. Thank you."

Say: "Divine Healing Intelligence, please heal and regenerate my uterus and all related organs to their maximum health, vitality, and well-being."

Unhealthy emotions to work with (page 171): Rejection 191, Judgment 188, Guilt 184, Sadness 193

Healthy emotions to work with (page 197): Recognition 204, Respect 205, Compassion 198, Forgiveness 200

Colors to work with (page 211): Yellow 221, Orange 216, Pink 217

## *Vagina*

### Possible Contributing Factors

Disconnected from feminine energy. Anger with a male, especially a partner. Holding on to feelings of shame and humiliation from the past. Feeling unattractive, unlovable, not good enough, rejected, or hurt by your partner. Overtired; too much giving to / mothering of everyone else leaving little personal time. Denying yourself pleasure. Fear of intimacy and of getting hurt. Rejection of self; frustration, wanting things to be different. Negative consequences from only financially motivated actions. Victim consciousness: *Poor me. They are doing this to me. I'm an innocent victim.*

### Remedy

Do you enjoy your sensuality? Are you connected to your feminine energy? Do you allow yourself time to do things that you enjoy, such as reading a book, going out with friends, having your hair done, or getting a massage? Do you enjoy making love, or do you carry feelings of shame, guilt, and a belief that your vagina is dirty?

Become aware of the amazing function of your vagina and reproductive system; appreciation of the system and of yourself heals those areas. List all the things you appreciate about being female, and the ways you could feel more feminine and enjoy your sensuality.

Imagine all the shame, guilt, anger, and "dirty" feelings being released from your vagina and reproductive system like dark rings of smoke.

Say: "Divine Healing Intelligence, please help me dissolve all anger with males, shame, guilt, rejection, denial of pleasure, frustration, hurt, and humiliation from my vagina, as well as all points of view, all patterns, and the positive and negative charges that contribute to this condition." Repeat the word "CLEAR" until you feel a shift occur.

Visualize your reproductive system filled with beautiful pink and magenta colors. Observe those colors as they regenerate your vagina and reproductive system, giving you an internal cleansing massage. Consider wearing pink or magenta underwear.

Say: "Divine Healing Intelligence, please help me feel more connected to my femininity; allow me to take time out for myself, to appreciate myself, and to rest. Allow me to forgive those who have hurt me and bring back the energy of excitement, pleasure, and sexuality. Thank you."

If you are open to exploring, remove your underwear, go to a mirror (or find a small mirror), and look at your vagina. Tell it how much you appreciate it; smile at it. Focus on relaxing and breathing into it. You might even want to touch different areas and become aware of how it feels. Give yourself an opportunity to get to know yourself intimately and to become comfortable with your sensuality.

Say: "Divine Healing Intelligence, please heal and regenerate my vagina and reproductive system to their maximum health, vitality, and well-being."

Unhealthy emotions to work with (page 171): Anger 173, Criticism 175, Judgment 188, Shame 193, Rejection 191, Feeling Overwhelmed 180
Healthy emotions to work with (page 197): Compassion 198, Recognition 204, Support 206, Love 203
Colors to work with (page 211): Orange 216, Green 213, Magenta 215, Pink 217

## Veins

### Possible Contributing Factors
Feeling cut off from a source of love and empowerment. Stuck, blocked. Stopping the struggle of life. Difficulty receiving pleasure and joy. Can't let go of old, outdated beliefs. Holding on to feelings of guilt, rejection, and humiliation. Experiencing fear of the future.

### Remedy
Think about what is happening in your life. Ask yourself:

*Where do I feel stuck in my life?*
*What thoughts, stories, and patterns keep repeating themselves?*

Say: "Divine Healing Intelligence, please help me dissolve all disempowerment, guilt, humiliation, blame, fear, and rejection from my veins, as well as all points of

117

view, all patterns, and the positive and negative charges that contribute to this condition. Repeat the word "CLEAR" until you feel a shift occur.

In order to create a healthy flow of energy in your body, you need to create a healthy flow of energy in your life. Become aware of the changes you need to make, and list these changes. Focus on the list every day, and make at least one change; then celebrate it.

After making this change, close your eyes and imagine beautiful indigo rays moving through all the veins in your body to dissolve any areas where energy is stuck. Then focus on the goals you are moving toward and visualize fulfilling these goals.

Say: "Divine Healing Intelligence, please help me reconnect to the source of love, well-being, and happiness. Allow me to move ahead with confidence into the future of my dreams. Thank you."

Say: "Divine Healing Intelligence, please heal and regenerate my veins to their maximum health, vitality, and well-being."

Unhealthy emotions to work with (page 171): Anger 173, Criticism 175, Judgment 188

Healthy emotions to work with (page 197): Love 203, Joy 203, Success 207, Freedom 201

Colors to work with (page 211): Indigo 214, Red 218, Blue 211

## *Wrists*

### Possible Contributing Factors
Feeling chained, stuck, overworked. Difficulty changing your mind; seeing other points of view; and letting go of the pain, stress, and fear that binds you. Needing to be right and in control.

### Remedy
If you wear watches or bracelets, do not wear them for several days to allow your wrists to relax.

Focus on your wrists. Do they feel free or do they feel stuck? Shake all stuckness from your wrists for thirty seconds, then relax for thirty seconds. Repeat this process five times.

Close your eyes and tune into your wrists. Are you wearing chains or shackles around them? What are these chains connected to? Is it your work, family, friends, or other commitments?

Say: "Divine Healing Intelligence, please help me dissolve all chains, stuckness, stress, fear, righteousness, and control from my wrists, as well as all points of view, all patterns, and the positive and negative charges that contribute to this condition." Repeat the word "CLEAR" until you feel a shift occur.

Visualize freeing your wrists from all chains or shackles. Then completely relax your wrists, and imagine bathing them in beautiful, warm, yellow liquid. Allow your wrists to become stronger.

Say: "Divine Healing Intelligence, please help me to free myself from all energies that bind me. Allow me to relax and become more peaceful, flexible, and tolerant. Thank you."

Say: "Divine Healing Intelligence, please heal and regenerate my wrists to their maximum strength, flexibility, and well-being."

Unhealthy emotions to work with (page 171): Stress 194, Fear 179, Control 174
Healthy emotions to work with (page 197): Flexibility and Movement 200,
  Relaxation 205, Freedom 201
Colors to work with (page 211): Yellow 221, Pink 217, Green 213

# II

# THE SECRET LANGUAGE OF PHYSICAL AILMENTS

In this section, you will find information about the emotional, mental, and energetic blocks that can contribute to a problem or disease in your body. The disease or disorder feeds on thoughts, feelings, or energies and continues to degenerate the body on a physical level. When you understand your blocks and limitations, you can begin to release them.

In the alphabetized list of ailments that follows, I have included emotions that I have found are commonly associated with each condition through my work. Remember to use the information in this section only as a guideline. I have listed examples of these emotions, but not every dense or destructive feeling or thought listed will relate to you. Tune into your body as you read the information, and notice which aspects of the condition or related emotions you react to. They will be the ones most relevant to your situation.

Often, just recognizing the thoughts, emotions, and attitudes that have contributed to the problem can initiate the healing process. This is because, when you have an awareness of the cause of the issue, you have choice. Choice gives you an opportunity to reflect on your life, become aware of what does not work, and do something different. Healing encompasses every aspect of your being, including your physical health and fitness, emotional well-being, mental attitude, energetic welfare, and spiritual strength. It is important to recognize that your body is not your enemy; it is a messenger that can help you to know yourself fully.

The following section offers you insights into issues you may need to confront and deal with in order to heal. Healing always means transformation. To heal, you need to change your thoughts, feelings, and actions from what does not work to what can and does work. You need to look at the problem your body is experiencing as a metaphorical representation of the challenges you are dealing with in your life.

Zelda came to see me because she had problems with her heart and wanted to find out what was the cause of her pain. When we looked at what was happening in Zelda's life, she began to see patterns emerging. Zelda held on to buried pain from the past, she was constantly stressed about her work, and she worried about people in her life. She lived alone, and felt isolated and lonely. She was also extremely self-critical of any little mistakes she made.

Once Zelda truly became aware of what she was doing to herself and how it was causing her heart disease, she began forgiving the people who had hurt her in the past, letting go of her buried pain. Zelda realized that her job was causing her a lot of unhappiness, and she quit. She also began to socialize more, relax, and do creative things that opened her heart. Rather than being so harsh with herself, she started using humor, laughing instead of beating herself up. Incredibly, her heart condition, which doctors had said was incurable, healed.

Ruth was the same way. Although she was unable to see me in person (she lived in a different city), we decided to organize a distance healing session. I learned that Ruth had a tumor growing on her pituitary gland, which was causing high levels of prolactin to enter her bloodstream. On the physical level, Ruth was experiencing severe headaches and visual problems. Although doctors recommended that she start taking heavy medication, she decided to try the natural approach.

I was able to share with Ruth the reasons for her tumor, and she was astounded at how accurately I read what was happening in her life. I recommended that she work with some of the exercises in this book, and after about six months I received a letter from her telling me how thrilled she was with her results. She told me that a few days after the healing treatment, her head felt much clearer, and she had not suffered one migraine since.

Ruth also went to a doctor for her yearly checkup. The doctor was astonished that the prolactin levels in her blood had reduced to near normal, a phenomenon he could not explain. Ruth felt that she had enormous proof of the power of her own self-healing ability.

I have traveled to many countries to teach my work and have received feedback from all over the world. A healthcare professional from Pakistan emailed me that he taught some processes from this book to twenty of his clients who had either high blood pressure or diabetes. Within three weeks all the participants reported that they had no more pain in their body, were no longer tired, and felt energetic. They did not feel thirsty or need to use the restroom as frequently. Among those who were helped by the processes, nine were on insulin and no longer required it.

My greatest desire is that the information and the processes in this book help you become vibrantly well and that you share this work, which is really "our work," with everyone you know. Your body is your teacher; it gives you opportunities to learn and expand. Once you have learned your lessons, it heals because there is no need to keep holding on to the pain any longer.

## List of Ailments

### A

**Abdominal Cramps**—Fear, anger, hurt. Allowing people to kick you in the gut. Blaming yourself and others. Stuck in a limited way of thinking and not seeing a way out of the situation. *See also* Cramps.

**Abscess**—Irritation, frustration, stagnation, swelling. Constantly replaying old hurts and criticisms. Negative outlook on life. Angry emotions that have festered and become inflamed. Suppressing something you do not want to look at, even though it keeps resurfacing. *See also* Anal Abscess.

**Accidents**—Feeling fearful, arrogant, rebellious. Belief in pain and punishment. Experiencing inner conflict. Feeling unbalanced, unfocused, confused. Overwhelmed by negative thoughts that replay endlessly.

**Acid Reflux**—Difficulty digesting life. Feeling uncomfortable with what you are seeing, feeling, hearing, and experiencing. Feeling irritated and frustrated about your inability to control what is happening around you. Guilt about the past. Feeling helpless about past choices. Resisting life rather than learning from your experiences.

**Acne**—Feeling uncomfortable in your own skin, insecure, unacceptable, rejected, not good enough, unworthy of love. Holding on to self-hatred. Trying to hurt and punish yourself for past mistakes. Controlling; demanding unrealistic perfection from self. Overly sensitive. *See also* Pimples (occasional).

**Acquired Immune Deficiency Syndrome (AIDS)**—Feeling guilty, wronged, disappointed, dirty. Sexual shame. Belief in inequality, injustice, and inferiority. Feeling defeated and not good enough, important, or worthy. Rejection of the self. Experiencing inner turmoil, struggle, and weakness.

**Addison's Disease**—Overly stressed. Worrying about everything and everyone, and taking everything to heart. Feeling anxious. Not allowing yourself to have a break or time out. Always busy trying to make something happen. Pushing against the current of your life. Feeling frustrated that things are not happening the way you want. Denying yourself fun, joy, and laughter.

**Addiction**—Seeking something outside yourself that can take the pain, stress, or anxiety away. Afraid that you are not a good person deep down inside. Running away from problems. Difficulty loving and accepting yourself.

**Adenoids**—Anger, family arguments, feeling left out or unloved. Trying to block out negativity and feelings of hopelessness.

**ADD/ADHD**—*See* Attention Deficit Hyperactivity Disorder.

**Aging (fear of)**—Fear of losing one's value. Belief in sickness and degeneration. Fear of change and transformation. Wanting things to stay the same rather than moving on and embracing new aspects of life.

**AIDS**—*See* Acquired Immune Deficiency Syndrome.

**Alcoholism**—Suppressed anger and hurt with nowhere to go. Self-punishment, boredom, stagnation, depression. In need of a way out. Too much thinking. Drowning in self-created problems, and pushing them away rather than dealing with them.

**Allergies**—Feeling annoyed and aggravated by other people. Giving away your power. Blaming people and events for your negative reactions. Obsession with people who have hurt you. Difficulty forgiving and seeing the blessing in this hurt. Allowing yourself to be controlled or manipulated by others, and then punishing them by withholding love and kindness. Not knowing how to create boundaries with others. *See also* Food Allergies/Sensitivities.

**Alzheimer's Disease**—Loss of power, inability to deal with life, too many suppressed emotions. Overwhelmed by life, wanting to run away to another time. Not wanting to remember or be present. Feeling lost and confused. Anxiety related to living life the way it is. Fear of dying and letting go.

**Amenorrhea (absence of menstruation)**—Feeling uncomfortable as a female. Carrying feelings of resentment about females, especially your mother. Feelings of abandonment; lack of nurturing and trust in your own power. Feeling weak, fragile, and vulnerable. Not knowing how to take care of yourself. Excessively exercising, over-dieting, abusing your body, and over-stressing.

**Amnesia**—Unsatisfied, unhappy, unfulfilled by life. Wiping out painful memories. Not wanting to deal with the past. Too many unresolved issues and suppressed emotions.

**Anemia**—Feeling exhausted. Loss of joy, creativity, and interest in life. Holding on to too many worries and concerns. Feeling like you're not good enough, not valuable. Invalidating yourself and your desires. Resisting life, and feeling limited and lost.

**Anal Abscess**—Resistance, fury, blame. Feeling ashamed about or victimized by something, and trying to hide it. Feeling guilty, bad, dirty. Trying to punish yourself and others. Wanting revenge. Feeling frustrated and overwhelmed by the feelings you are trying not to feel. *See also* Abscess.

**Anal Bleeding**—Pushing too hard. Forcing things to happen rather than allowing them to happen. Refusing to deal with unresolved issues. Wanting things your own way. Fear of loss. Resisting change. Anger, frustration, unhappiness about what is happening in your life. Difficulty with boundaries. Trying to control the uncontrollable.

**Aneurysm**—Feeling overwhelmed, that life is too hard, that nothing is working. Difficulty asking for support. Feeling that a situation has gone too far and there is no turning back. Needing to get out of a situation in any way possible. Working yourself to death. Carrying too many problems and responsibilities. Stubborn.

**Angina**—Stress, frustration, fear of the future. Difficulty showing emotion, especially love. Feeling closed off from life; angry, judgmental. Feeling that life is unjust.

**Anorexia**—Trying to control your life by denying yourself nourishment. Extreme anger, hatred, and rejection of self. Belief in self-punishment. An unhappy childhood, painful family life. Denial of joy and fun. Feeling like you don't belong. Inability to communicate and deal with your fears. Wasting away.

**Anosmia**—*See* Smell (loss of).

**Anxiety**—Thinking about the past and the future, and not trusting the flow of life. Feeling insecure, unsupported, and helpless to change your situation. Focusing on negativity and limitation, and allowing yourself to wallow in fear.

**Appendicitis**—Loss of power. Feeling like you can't get what you want. Denial of life. Feeling dejected, fearful, angry, and uninspired.

**Arthritis**—Holding on to anger and resentment from the past. Carrying guilt, remorse, and shame. Difficulty forgiving yourself and others. Complaining about life. Worrying but not wanting to make changes. Feeling stuck and limited.

**Asperger Syndrome**—Difficulty fitting in. Feeling like no one understands or relates to you. A sense of isolation, loneliness, and separation. Fear of not being accepted or liked. Feeling uncomfortable with people, not knowing how to communicate your feelings. Seeming aggressive and forceful when all you really desire is attention, love, and understanding.

**Asthma**—Trying too hard to please others. Wanting to be perfect. Difficulty saying no, standing up for yourself, and expressing how you feel. Pushing yourself to the limit until you feel exhausted and out of breath. Feeling weak, anxious, and disempowered. Allowing others to control you. Feeling hurt, stuck, caged.

**Astigmatism**—*See under* Eye Conditions.

**Atherosclerosis (hardening of the arteries)**—Judging, criticizing, condemning. Losing touch with your feelings and connection with your heart. Following your head rather than your heart. Fear of loving yourself and others. Seeing yourself in a negative light. Keeping people at a distance. Nursing old hurts. Being hard on yourself and others.

**Athlete's Foot**—Irritation, anger, and frustration, as if someone or something has gotten under your skin. Feeling like you are being held back. Unresolved family anger. Feeling unaccepted, blocked, and confused.

**Attention Deficit Hyperactivity Disorder (ADHD/ADD)**—Difficulty concentrating or paying attention. Boredom, frustration, aggression. Not knowing how to share or communicate your feelings. Feeling trapped, forced to do what you don't want to do and what does not interest you.

**Autism**—Feeling imprisoned inside a limited world and frustrated by your dependence on others. A sense of being shut out and looked down on. Desire to rise beyond, and show your creativity and genius. Fearful of being laughed at, cast out, or humiliated. Not knowing how to get in touch with your own intuition.

## B

**Bacterial Infection**—Feeling weak, easily affected by others, needy. Desiring attention at any cost. Feeling infuriated, frustrated, irritated. Keeping things inside instead of sharing, letting go, and creating change.

**Balance (loss of)**—Feeling unstable. Difficulty getting your bearings. Feeling like you are being pulled in different directions, creating confusion and scattered thinking.

**Baldness**—Too much stress and fear of the future. Difficulty trusting. Trying to manipulate and control events. Living on adrenaline and frustration. Difficulty handling disappointment, wanting to rip your hair out with frustration. *See also* Gray Hair *and* Hair Loss.

**Bedwetting**—Afraid of authority. Loss of control; feelings of uncertainty. Fear of punishment.

**Belching**—*See* Burping.

**Bell's Palsy**—Resisting a challenging situation or person. Too much stress. Stuckness. Numbing your feelings. Refusing to listen to others or to see a situation in a different way. Feeling weak, defeated, trapped. Worrying about how others see you. Wearing masks.

**Bipolar Disorder (Manic Depression)**—Extreme imbalance, stress, trauma. A possible shock that occurred in childhood, such as a death in the family, divorce, an accident, or seeing a close friend or member of the family endure an incurable illness. Feeling out of place. Wanting to be somewhere that you are not. Feeling controlled and dominated, and wanting to break free. Fear that something bad or dark is living inside you that you have no control over. A lot of internal aggression and frustration that you don't know how to handle.

**Birth Defects**—Karmic decision to come into this life to learn lessons of humility and love. Carrying intense stress and anxiety from the womb in relation to parents.

**Blacking Out**—Loss of balance. Feeling overwhelmed by life; needing to find a way out. Too much pressure, anxiety, trauma.

**Bladder Cancer**—Uncomfortable with what you are feeling or doing in your life. Guilt about past or present actions. Internal conflict. A need for boundaries and your own space. Feeling angry or pissed off with a person close to you, but burying these feelings instead of expressing them. A deep sense of unresolved sadness. *See also* Cancer.

**Bleeding**—Self-sabotage; holding on to the belief that you deserve to be punished and to experience pain. Too much focus on negativity and why things are not working instead of how they can work. Feeling that you need to struggle and suffer to achieve.

**Bleeding Gums**—Feeling unsure of yourself. Difficulty asking for help. Feeling unsupported. Wanting things yesterday. Refusing to change. Extremely demanding of yourself and others. Neglecting your body.

**Blepharitis (eyelid inflammation)**—*See under* Eye Conditions.

**Blindness**—Not wanting to see what is going on around you. Feeling intimidated by life and people. Resisting what you don't like. Turning a blind eye to things you don't want to see. A need to look within and to find a different reality, as the outer one is too painful. *See also* Color Blindness *under* Eye Conditions.

**Blisters**—Pushing past your limits. Not listening to or honoring your body. Too caught up in stresses and worries of the outside world.

**Bloated**—Holding on to anger; trying to find someone to blame; feeling like a victim, helpless and hopeless. Worrying too much and holding on to fear. Constant self-doubt and self-sabotage. Buying into the belief that you are not good enough.

**Blood Clotting**—Blocking creativity and energy flow, resisting life. Too focused on limitations. Lack of belief in self. Inner turmoil, deep disappointment, regret.

**Blood Pressure**—*See* Hypertension *and* Hypotension.

**Body Odor**—Feeling uncomfortable, rejected by others, mocked, unaccepted. Fear of others and their judgment of you. Deep-seated self-criticism and self-loathing.

**Boils**—Blood-boiling anger that has been carefully controlled. Feeling uncomfortable about what you are doing or have to do. Deep-seated resentment and bitterness about your lot in life. Feelings of unfairness and injustice. Tendency to blame others.

**Bone Breaks**—Pushing yourself beyond your limit. Overworking. Trying to get out of a difficult situation. Belief in self-punishment—that you deserve to be abused, either mentally, emotionally, or physically. Not honoring your word. Reaching your breaking point.

**Bone Cancer**—Deep rage, trauma, and fear. Holding on to deep-seated pain and resentment from the past. Unable to hold on to the pain and pressure anymore. Feeling fragile. Struggling to survive. Constant attack on self. Too many burdens and unresolved issues that are eating away at you. *See also* Cancer.

**Bone Deformity**—Going against what you believe. Constantly doing things that others want you to do. Pushing your dreams or goals aside. Feeling devastated by the events of your life. Deep betrayal and loss of hope. Stuck in a pattern of continuous struggle.

**Bone Marrow Conditions**—Loss of faith. Disappointment in self and others. Carrying feelings of failure and insecurity. Fear of moving forward and doing things on your own. Hiding your talents and abilities from others, thus hindering any potential success. Too clingy and needy of others' approval. *See also* Inflammation *and* Osteomyelitis (bone and bone marrow inflammation).

**Bone Weakness**—Lack of support. Giving away your power. Feeling weak, unsure, limited. Buying into the judgment and criticism of others. Feeling controlled, unprotected, defenseless, weary. Carrying a lot of stress and worry in your bones. Feeling isolated and abandoned, like you have no one to rely on. A deep, internal neediness to be taken care of.

**Brain Tumor**—In conflict with yourself. Surrounded by negativity and instability. Blaming yourself for mistakes of the past. Feeling trapped or out of control without knowing how to change.

**Breast Cancer**—Inability to nurture yourself because you take on everybody else's problems. Feeling guilty and wronged. Too much worry and apprehension. Lack of self-confidence and love. Feeling like a victim. *See also* Cancer.

**Breast Cyst/Lump**—Holding on to past hurts and regretting past decisions. Sadness about how things have turned out, lost dreams. Feeling unfulfilled by life. Difficulty asking for help. Not knowing how to say no. A lack of nurturing and comfort. Feeling unsupported by life and people. *See also* Cancer *and* Cyst.

**Breast Feeding (loss of)**—Feeling inadequate. Blaming yourself for challenges you are experiencing. Extremely stressed and overwhelmed by the responsibility of being a mother. Trying to control circumstances and feeling disempowered.

**Breath (bad)**—Feeling angry; wanting to keep others away. Feeling unacceptable, rejected, and uncomfortable. Difficulty fitting in.

**Bronchitis**—Feeling too much pressure. Conflict and anger in the family, which leads to irritation with people close to you. Blaming others for what you can't fix or control. Needing time out and time to yourself. Feeling a lack of appreciation and love. Pushing people away.

**Bruising**—Reacting to life in an aggravated way. Feeling a lack of clarity and making silly mistakes for which you blame yourself. Self-punishment.

**Bulimia**—Difficulty receiving love and nourishment. Constant self-criticism, guilt, and self-sabotage. Trying to control situations. Using food to push problems away instead of facing them.

**Bunion**—Following the wrong direction in life. Making decisions that have limited your growth and expansion. Fear of change. Lack of belief in your ability to create and become successful.

**Burnout**—Overcommitting and pushing yourself too hard, not knowing when to stop. Perfectionism. Resisting different points of view. Forcing things to happen. Difficulty saying no. Putting others' needs before your own. Stubbornness; refusing to listen to your body and recognize your value. An attitude that nothing is ever enough. *See also* Burns.

**Burns**—Feeling burned out or tired. Lack of clarity. Loss of direction. Anger with people who refuse to listen to you or to follow your advice. Impatience. *See also* Burnout.

**Burping**—Lack of freedom. Feeling like decisions have been taken away from you. Feeling challenged in a relationship that feels heavy and unyielding. Trying to push things away. Limiting what you allow into your life. Difficulty receiving great things into your life. Feeling overwhelmed, like you have too much to handle all at once.

**Bursitis**—Feeling stuck in a pattern. Difficulty getting out of your comfort zone. Overwhelmed by fear and all there is to do in order to move forward. Feeling bored, dissatisfied, angry, and uninspired. Carrying an internal conflict that is eating away at you. Loss of direction. Feeling powerless.

# C

**Callus Formation**—Resisting your feelings. Becoming hard. Getting stuck in a limited perspective. Fear of trusting your instincts and taking empowering action. Great at giving good advice to others but not at taking any yourself.

**Cancer**—Feeling limited, angry, fearful, out of control. Carrying wounds from the past. Not feeling good enough, shrinking inside and attacking yourself from within. Feeling like guilt, grief, and uncertainty are eating away at your body. On guard, never able to relax and let go. Often pushing yourself to do more than you can handle. Trying to please others and constantly seeking approval. *See also* Bladder Cancer, Bone Cancer, Breast Cancer, Breast Cyst/Lump, Cervical Cancer, Leukemia, Lung Cancer, Lymphoma, Ovarian Cancer, Prostate Cancer, *and* Skin Cancer.

**Candida**—Self-doubt. Feeling scattered, hazy, frazzled, stressed, trapped. Frustrated with your partner, blaming your partner or someone close to you. Feeling angry that you aren't getting what you want, but not wanting to change or to take positive action. Difficulty trusting and confiding in people.

**Canker Sores**—Insecurity. Constant self-doubt and distrust of your capacities. Holding back and not speaking up. Allowing opportunities to pass you by. Feeling regret and frustration.

**Carpal Tunnel Syndrome**—Wanting to be numb. Doing what you don't want to do. Blocking the energy flow in your life. Holding on to grief and sadness from the past. Struggling; too much strain and difficulty. Feeling like you can't handle something.

**Car Sickness**—Fear of being out of control. Belief that you have no choice. Feeling trapped and confused.

**Cataracts**—*See under* Eye Conditions.

**Cavities**—Self neglect. Anger. Resisting forgiveness of those who have hurt you. Too serious about life. Carrying shame. Critical of self and others. Stubbornness, aggression, wanting things your own way. Lacking sweetness, inspiration, and gentleness.

**Cellulite**—Feeling unbalanced, up and down. Belief that life is tough and fraught with many obstacles. Thinking that the older you get, the more challenges you have to face. Resisting life and putting issues on the back burner, rather than dealing with them in the present.

**Cerebral Palsy**—Deep discomfort with life. Feeling, stuck and confined, unable to express yourself. Cannot comfortably inhabit the body you were given; it is beyond your control. From birth, feeling overwhelmed. The belief that life is a struggle, uncontrollable and unpredictable.

**Cervical Cancer**—Out of flow with life. Resisting your femininity. Feeling disrespected as a woman. Feeling unwanted, lacking in affection, sexually conflicted. Feeling frustrated because of a lack of commitment or attention in a relationship. Feeling ignored, unimportant, useless, empty, cheated. *See also* Cancer.

**Chest Congestion**—Holding back, feeling blocked. Difficulty communicating and asking for what you want. Allowing others to dictate you, and then feeling angry and resentful toward them.

**Chicken Pox**—Feeling irritated, unappreciated, and unnoticed. Needing love and attention, and time out to rest. Feeling unsettled and agitated, like you don't belong. Experiencing disappointment and feeling let down.

**Childhood Diseases**—Need for attention and love. Feeling left out, upset, not sure how to deal with life. Fearful, especially if parents fought or still fight. Holding on to guilt and making yourself sick by taking on your parents' worries. Belief in punishment for bad behavior. Feeling unworthy and undeserving of love and affection. Inner battle.

**Chills**—Processing an experience or situation that is beyond your comfort zone. Feeling exposed, vulnerable, unprotected. Restricted, frozen. Not sure what step to take next. Internal confusion and fear of making the wrong decisions.

**Chlamydia**—Feeling ashamed, irritated, taken advantage of. Allowing people to feed off you like parasites. Feeling angry, rejected, lonely, and undervalued. Constantly wondering what is wrong with you. Uncomfortable with your body and your sexuality.

**Cholesterol**—Feeling vulnerable and in need of protection. Keeping secrets; continually feeling under threat and ready to fight. Constantly on guard, expecting something bad to happen. Holding on to pain and limitation from the past in order to cushion yourself for the next blow. Lack of joy, fun, and laughter. Carrying too much nervous energy and too easily irritated.

**Chronic Illness**—Feeling stuck, refusing to change. Receiving attention and support from people that you are afraid you would lose if you got better. Comfortable with not being well, self-pitying, holding on to victim consciousness, settling for your lot in life. Choosing to give up or not participate because life is too scary and demanding.

**Chronic Fatigue Syndrome**—Resisting life. Not knowing how to say no. Frustrated about constantly having to do what you don't want to do. Wishing you were somewhere else. Belief that life is heavy and hard, and that you have to toil to get anywhere. Pushing past your limits. Feeling stuck. Ignoring your body, intuition, and creativity. Thinking that someone else is right and has the answers. Giving away your power.

**Circulation Problems**—Feeling stuck, restricted, held back, like you have been going round and round in circles with no change. Allowing others to make important decisions and then blaming them when things go wrong. Fear of taking risks. Doing things the way you were taught rather than trying new things.

**Claustrophobia**—Feeling anxious, obsessive, worried, stuck, imprisoned in your own reality. Needing to control everything and everyone, and feeling out of control. Trying hard to make everything perfect but failing. Carrying a lot of suppressed anger and disappointment.

**Cluster Headache**—Frustrated, critical, angry. Suspecting people are backstabbing you. Guarded. Disappointed in yourself and others. Thinking too much. Wanting to stand up for yourself but not knowing how. Feeling attacked and criticized from all directions. Too much going on. Not knowing when to stop. Lack of self-belief. *See also* Headache, Migraine.

**Celiac Disease**—Feeling overly sensitive, easily hurt, and irritated. Difficulty standing up for yourself. Constantly focusing on what's wrong rather than what's right. Difficulty dealing with criticism.

**Cold (common)**—Scattered; too much to do, too many responsibilities, too much pressure to perform. Refusing to listen to your body and slow down. Feeling overwhelmed, overworked, and worn out. In need of some time to yourself. Confused about what choices to make. *See also* Influenza.

**Cold Sore**—Feeling deprived, like you are not getting what you want. Difficulty communicating your desires because of fear of rejection or of not being liked. Feeling uncomfortable, disappointed, and angry. Allowing others to control and manipulate you, then feeling let down, frustrated, and disillusioned.

**Colic**—Feeling scared, unsupported, irritated, impatient. In need of attention and love.

**Colitis**—Difficulty digesting life. Apprehension; suppressing painful emotions instead of dealing with them. A cry for help. Feeling defeated and worthless. Wanting to give up or give in. Feeling that it's all too much to cope with. Difficulty seeing other people's points of view. Great need for approval and to be right.

**Color Blindness**—*See under* Eye Conditions.

**Coma**—Not wanting to be here. Fear of the future. Feeling unable to cope with life as it is. Needing to escape or to get out of a situation.

**Compulsive Eating**—Struggling with destructive emotions that you push down or shut out. Covering your feelings and the messages your body is trying to give you. Afraid that allowing yourself to feel will make you depressed or in danger of exploding, or make everything fall apart. Feeling guilt and shame. Needing to control. Fear of failure. Trying to fill an internal void.

**Conjunctivitis**—*See under* Eye Conditions.

**Constipation**—Feeling closed off, holding back, stuck in an old way of thinking. Refusing to make decisions, to see other people's points of view, or to make changes. Trying to convince others that you are right, that you know better; a "my way or the highway" attitude. Holding on to old fear and anger. In some cases, acting extremely selfish, demanding, and self-obsessed, exhibiting childish traits. Feeling unloved, undervalued, and unappreciated. Constantly worrying about the future.

**Convulsions**—Internal conflict, resistance, and upheaval. Passive aggression. Dissatisfaction, which leads to internal anger and violence. Trying hard to suppress and control what you consider to be your dark side.

**Coronary Thrombosis**—Stopping the flow of life. Closing your heart to others. Not feeling good enough or worthy of love. Holding on to a belief that you are useless. Thinking nobody cares. Feeling betrayed by others, allowing pain and grief to block the flow of blood to your heart. Experiencing a lack of joy and zest for life.

**Corn**—Feeling uneasy about the future. Fear of moving forward. Resisting the natural flow of life. Fear of failure. Desperately trying to please others in order to get approval.

**Cough**—Resistant to making a necessary change in your life. Feeling overwhelmed by worries, anxieties, and stresses. Trying to meddle in other people's lives, focusing on fixing their issues instead of dealing with your own to divert attention from yourself. Easily irritated by people, especially those close to you. Self-critical. Easily influenced by others.

**Cramps**—Too much stress and tension. Overwhelmed by fear and struggle. Holding on to the belief that life is too hard. Inability to relax and let go. Feeling restless and tired. Overly demanding, wanting things right away. Frustrated, irritated, and discouraged. *See also* Abdominal Cramps.

**Crohn's Disease**—Negative attitude and criticism, constant self-abuse. A tendency to see life from a gloomy or cynical perspective. Trying to suppress rather than allowing to feel uncomfortable feelings. Constantly hiding your sensitivity; pretending to be confident and undisturbed by other people's comments while feeling sick on the inside. A tendency to blame others and feel like a victim.

**Cross-Eyed (eyes deviate inward)**—*See* Esotropia *under* Eye Conditions.

**Crying**—Allowing yourself to let go of tension and old stresses. An opportunity to see life from a different point of view. Extremely healing if suppressed feelings get acknowledged and are then let go. Washing out your insides to make room for insights. In some cases, shedding tears of joy.

**Cushing's Syndrome**—Constant self-sabotage. Weighed down by problems and issues you don't know how to resolve. Overwhelmed by life. Feeling thin-skinned, like you are unable to handle even the smallest setbacks without falling into a heap. Belief that everything is hard and nobody can help.

**Cyst**—Unfulfilled dreams. Holding on to regrets, which prevent you from moving forward. Fear of being hurt and taken advantage of. Holding on to disappointments and failures from the past. Buying into fears and false ideas. Allowing doubts and limitations to dominate your life. *See also* Breast Cyst/Lump, Fibroid Tumor/Cyst, *and* Ovarian Cyst.

**Cystic Fibrosis**—Belief that life is too complicated. Feeling like you can't thrive. Nothing works for you, and nobody understands or supports you. Thinking that you are the victim. Holding on to resentment, anger, and the belief that there is something wrong with you—that you're a mistake and nobody wants you.

# D

**Dandruff**—Too much stress; too many things to do and people to please. Things crumbling in your life. In constant overdrive, which has dried up your energy and creativity.

**Deafness**—Not liking what you are hearing. Overwhelmed by the negativity. Blocking your ears. Constantly saying or thinking, *I don't want to hear it.* Feeling rejected and rejecting others. Feeling like a victim. Thinking that what you say or communicate is not important and that people don't want to hear you. Being stubborn, inflexible, or controlling. *See also* Earache.

**Death (fear of)**—Attached to your body and physical life. Unprepared to move into your next phase as a spirit; lack of trust, faith. Feeling incomplete with life.

**Dementia**—*See* Alzheimer's Disease.

**Depression**—Pressure to survive. Feeling overwhelmed, hopeless, disappointed, and disillusioned. Wanting someone to save you. Suppressed anger and resentment. Feeling and acting like a victim. Blaming others for what is not working in your life. Feeling unmotivated and uninspired. Can't be bothered to do anything. Stuck in an old story that's only getting gloomier.

**Depression (postnatal)**—Feelings of separation, abandonment, emptiness. Difficulty coping with extra responsibilities. Overwhelmed, isolated, lonely, sad. Not feeling good enough. Lack of trust and belief in your capacities. Buying into self-destructive thoughts.

**Dermatitis**—Irritated, unsatisfied, frustrated. Feeling anger inside that's being pushed through the skin. Constant criticism and judgment of self and others. Feeling uncomfortable in your own skin, unsure of yourself. Experiencing negative and depressing thoughts and feelings about yourself.

**Diabetes, Type 1**—Needing sweetness, attention, love, and care. Feeling insecure, unsure of yourself, overly needy, and reliant on others. Self-centered and focused on your inadequacies. Wanting to appear indispensable to others. Listening to and surrounding yourself with too much negativity.

**Diabetes, Type 2**—Fear of fully participating in life. Great need for control and to know things. Deep need for attention and approval. A constant craving for love paired with a belief that you are unworthy or undeserving. Deep-seated guilt. Belief that you have to struggle to survive. Often losing yourself in relationships. Constant need for sweetness to mask feelings of weakness, limitation, and the belief that there is not enough. Stuck in your own world of limitation and lack.

**Diarrhea**—Feeling uncomfortable with decisions you have made. Unsure how to ask for help. Feeling helpless, lost, unsupported, insecure, and confused. Experiencing fear and apprehension. *See also* Dysentery.

**Diplopia**—*See under* Eye Conditions.

**Diverticulitis (inflammation of the intestinal wall)**—Holding back, suppressing your feelings, hiding secrets. Feeling bound and constrained. Difficulty releasing fear and stress, and letting go. Feeling that you have no choice and just have to deal with your lot in life. Continuous self-sabotage. Often wanting to give up, thinking, *What is the point of trying when it all falls apart anyway? See also* Inflammation.

**Dizziness**—Feeling overloaded, unstable, and off balance, like you can't get your bearings. Things always seeming different from what you want or expect. Feeling unsafe, scattered, burdened. Wanting to be somewhere other than where you are. Difficulty accepting things as they are. Going round and round in circles, not sure which direction to take or changes to make.

**Double Vision**—*See* Diplopia *under* Eye Conditions.

**Down Syndrome**—A choice to incarnate and experience spontaneity, internal freedom, sensitivity, and natural emotions. Here to teach people to be free of societal pressure. Children with Down syndrome can teach parents unconditional love, openness, and emotional freedom. Because this syndrome can make a person hide, depend on others, and bring up feelings of powerlessness, aggression, lack of control, and anxiety, it is important that these children experience the safety, love, and the affection they desire.

**Dreams**—Repressed thoughts, ideas, and experiences enabling you to receive insights, visions, ideas, new perspectives, and solutions to unresolved issues. Often predictive, problem solving, creative, and releasing.

**Drug Addiction**—Needing a hit of something to save you, to take away the pain, and to help you cope. Escape from life's difficulties. Inability to cope or to get help. Fear of the unknown.

**Duodenal Problems**—Difficulty letting go of outdated ways of thinking, living, and communicating. So much going on that you don't know how to process and try to push away. Fear of the future and what it may bring.

**Dysentery**—Inability to take the way things are happening anymore. The body rebelling. Need for something to change fast. Losing touch with your essential nature and inner knowing, and forgetting how to make empowering decisions. Internal powerlessness, rage, resentment, and blame. *See also* Diarrhea.

**Dyslexia**—Feeling pushed to perform and to please people. Shamed, humiliated, and embarrassed for not living up to your parents' and teachers' expectations and for your lack of original ideas. Wanting to do things your way. Desire to communicate on a deep, soulful level, which is often misunderstood by others.

## E

**Earache**—Feeling judged and judging others. Not listening to your own insight and wisdom. Not wanting to hear what is being said, trying to block other people out. Feeling like others want to control you. Blame, frustration, anger, misunderstanding, arguments. Refusing to change your mind or perspective. Feeling ignored, unnoticed, resentful, unsteady. *See also* Deafness.

**Eclampsia (seizures/convulsions during pregnancy)**—Feeling constricted, imprisoned, stuck. Unsure how to handle the future. Fear of the extra responsibilities. Feeling insecure, unsafe, anxious, threatened. Fear of not being a good mother and having the ability to provide for your baby. Ill at ease about losing your freedom and sense of self. Feeling powerless about the future.

**Eczema**—Feeling unaccepted, needing to hide and suppress your feelings. Aggravated by your experiences with others. Erupting with anger when you don't get your way. Holding your breath. Experiencing a sense of stagnation.

**Edema**—Holding on to hurts from the past. Trying to control and suppress overflowing emotion. Hiding from, rather than confronting, challenges. Anxiety, quelled anger, procrastination, vulnerability, lack of confidence. Hesitation in moving forward.

**Emphysema**—Life feels like a struggle. Belief in hardness and limitation. Feeling like a victim, left out and rejected. Experiencing a sense of dread, like something bad is going to happen. Lack of joy. Too much thinking. Difficulty living in the moment. Feeling worn out by stress and worry.

**Encephalitis (viral)**—Surrounded by an overwhelming amount of cynicism and hardship. Too much thinking, which leads to more negativity and frustration. Don't know which way to turn. Feeling overwhelmed, oversensitive, and easily affected by your environment. Desire to run away and hide but with nowhere to go. Too much happening. Feeling attacked, invaded, criticized, judged, and condemned.

**Endometriosis**—Feeling inadequate and unacceptable. Rejecting the feminine aspect of yourself. Feeling depleted, unsupported, ungrounded. Holding on to feelings of rejection from others, especially men. Devaluing and dishonoring yourself. Denying yourself love and appreciation.

**Epilepsy**—Feeling attacked, criticized, and condemned to a certain fate. Out of balance with life. Feeling neglected, mistreated, abandoned, unwanted, violated. Belief that something is wrong with you.

**Epstein-Barr**—Oversensitive, not feeling good enough, lacking confidence, constantly changing your mind. Carrying a lot of suppressed energy. Uncontrollable aggression toward people who are close to you. Feeling guilty about your incapacity to stick to one thing. Disconnected from who you truly are. Focusing on other people's dreams instead of your own.

**Esotropia (eyes deviated inward)**—*See under* Eye Conditions.

**Exotropia (eyes deviated outward)**—*See under* Eye Conditions.

**Eye Conditions**

*Astigmatism*—A distorted view of life. Arguing with reality, wanting things to be different. Unable to accept yourself or your life experience. Holding on to feelings of rejection.

*Blepharitis (eyelid inflammation)*—Frustration, anger, internal conflict. Difficulty protecting and backing yourself. Doubting; changing your mind according to what you see instead of what you feel and know. *See also* Inflammation.

*Cataracts*—Nothing is clear; future seems blurry. Feeling like there's little hope of change, as though you are doomed to a gloomy existence. Burdened by life. Losing faith.

*Conjunctivitis*—Feeling irritated by what you are seeing. Trying to resist or block out what is happening in your life. Fear of the future. Feeling inadequate and believing that others see you as a failure. Feeling agitated and frustrated.

*Color Blindness*—Blocking, changing, refusing to see colors that incite horror or cause you stress, often from a shock or trauma in childhood that became associated with these particular colors. *See also* Blindness.

*Diplopia (double vision)*—Long-standing stress. Blurry and lacking clarity. Fear or internal conflict, which leads to seeing more than one possibility. Difficulty making decisions. Regrets. Unsure what to do. Feeling threatened. Alert and watchful of potential danger.

*Esotropia (eyes deviated inward)*—Believing what you are seeing is forbidden. Guilt. Fear of punishment for doing something bad or wrong. Feeling of impending danger. Thinking that someone is out to get you. Constantly stressed and on guard. Feeling "less than" in the eyes of others. Trying to push others out of your field of vision.

*Exotropia (eyes deviated outward)*—Bored, disinterested in what is occurring in your immediate environment; spaced out and overwhelmed. Needing to tune within and discover your unique abilities. Resisting what is being told to you. Overtired, frustrated, pushed, strained.

*Farsightedness*—Disappointment in the past; disillusionment and difficulties in dealing with the present.

*Glaucoma*—Feeling boxed in and under pressure, which is overwhelming, and mentally and emotionally exhausting. Pressure blocking your vision of the future. Difficulty forgiving others and letting go of blockages.

*Keratitis (cornea inflammation)*—Feeling powerless. Internal rage, irritation, and deep sadness. Extreme stress, anxiety, and fear of opening up to people. Deeply disappointed by your experiences and horrified by what you have seen. Distrusting of people or even yourself. Feeling like you have seen enough. Deep desire to see something different than what is in front of you. Holding self back because of past hurt. *See also* Inflammation.

*Nearsightedness*—Apprehension. Doubting your ability to cope with the future and feeling overwhelmed.

*Sty*—Feeling stuck, fearful, confused, disorientated. Carrying anger and resentment from the past. Constantly invalidating yourself and abandoning your resolutions. Inability to make up your mind.

## F

**Fainting**—Feeling overwhelmed by fear, that too much is going on. Inability to cope. Looking for a way out. Feeling tired and stressed.

**Farsightedness**—*See under* Eye Conditions.

**Fat**—Feeling vulnerable, inadequate, unattractive, depressed. Overeating to push down feelings. Belief that if you are bigger, you will be able to protect yourself from pain. Feeling stuck, unmotivated, unbalanced. Holding on to pain and resentment from the past. Punishing yourself with food. Trying to push away people and keep them at a distance. Constantly procrastinating, feeling unworthy of having good things in your life. *See also* Obesity *and* Overweight.

**Fatigue**—Stress, resistance, struggle, limitation. Fighting to get things done. Overworking and pushing yourself beyond your limit. Bored and frustrated with your life. Drained by your commitments.

**Fertility (difficulty conceiving)**—Fear of losing your freedom. Not feeling supported. Unsure if you will make a good parent. Limited ideas about parenthood. Unresolved issues from your own childhood. Blocking the process by being desperate to conceive. Feeling angry, resentful, and hurt that you can't, or fearful that you may not be able to. Feeling jealous and irritated that other people have children and you don't. Self criticism, lack of fun, not trusting life, not allowing yourself to enjoy your connections with children.

**Fever**—Inner turmoil, exhaustion, fragility. Feeling out of balance, undermined, fired up, angry. Taking on too much responsibility. Belief that situations have been dealt with unfairly.

**Fibroid Tumor/Cyst**—Holding on to hurts and regrets from the past. Secretly wanting revenge. Feeling disempowered and victimized, forced into things you don't want to do. Nursing disappointments and failures from the past. *See also* Cyst.

**Fibromyalgia**—Feeling unwanted, knocked down by life's challenges; overstressed. Lacking the strength to get up and keep going. Too much to do, and not enough time and energy to do it. Life feels like a fight. Feeling stuck, resistant to growth, movement, and exploration. Overflowing with sadness, regret, guilt, and worry. Feeling depressed, suppressed, and on guard.

**Flatulence**—Holding back. Feeling uncomfortable. Inability to express your emotions clearly. Resistant to change.

**Flu**—*See* Influenza.

**Food Allergies/Sensitivities**—Feeling irritated by what is happening around you. Extremely sensitive to other people's behaviors and beliefs about you. Feeling frustrated that your discomforts with life have not been heard and solved. Resisting life. Too focused on what you like and don't like. Not allowing full expression of who you are. *See also* Allergies.

**Frigidity**—Hurting, rejected, and angry. Feeling bound, unhappy, unbalanced, un-grounded, and disconnected from sensuality. Carrying judgments about sex. Denial of joy and pleasure. Disconnection from your body. Fear of domination. Need to control.

**Frozen Shoulder**—Suppressing your feelings. Experiencing too much strain, stress, and worry. Not dealing with your challenges by "numbing" them. Feeling stuck, trying to control rather than allow. Fear of the future. Wanting to give up. Feeling like a failure. Engulfed by problems. Unsure how to heal your pain and sadness. Represents frozen tears.

**Fungus**—Irritation, lack of boundaries; allowing people to get under your skin and feed off your energy. Buying into concepts that are stale and moldy. Doing things you disagree with. Feeling manipulated or forced into situations you don't want to be in. Family secrets, which may be festering beneath your skin or nails.

## G

**Gallstones**—Grief that has hardened. Feelings of resentment, irritability, depression. Disappointment about your achievement in the world. Either holding back or exploding with anger. Feeling wounded and trying to find someone to blame for your pain and suffering. Difficulty forgiving.

**Gangrene**—Feeling like life is not worth living. Festering negativity, constant complaining, self-loathing. Resisting life, feeling cut off from joy. Withering life force. Self-destruction.

**Gastritis**—Inability to handle constant bickering, fear, frustration, and negativity. Feeling rejected, disappointed, sad. So much going on that you can't digest life's challenges and difficulties. Easily irritated, feeling uncertain of yourself and the future.

**Gastrointestinal Ulcer**—*See* Ulcer (gastrointestinal).

**Genital Herpes**—Attack on yourself. Feeling rejected, abandoned, unworthy, and unlovable. Carrying enormous guilt about sexuality. Anger about how you have been treated. Belief that you are sinful or need to be punished. Feeling dirty, ashamed, humiliated, dishonored, and violated.

**Gingivitis**—Feeling irritated, stirred up, ungrounded, vulnerable, easily hurt. Carrying anger, shame, a sense of degradation. Rotten attitude about life. Procrastination. Always feeling like there is not enough time for yourself.

**Glandular Fever**—A "can't be bothered" attitude. Indecision, confusion, chaos. Worn out, disheartened. Difficulty communicating. Unable to say what you want. Allowing other people to push you around and drain your energy. Lack of boundaries.

**Glaucoma**—*See under* Eye Conditions.

**Gluten Intolerance**—Difficulty digesting and assimilating important events in your life, especially in childhood. Disliking parts of yourself. Trying to avoid confrontation at all costs. Neglecting yourself and what you feel. Feeling stuck, imprisoned, caged in your life.

**Goiter**—Scared to say what you really feel and live your life the way you want to. Always hiding and trying to please people, especially your family. Fear of being abused, criticized, or rejected for your choices. Shutting yourself out from your creativity and manifestation abilities. Feeling that you should just settle instead of asking for what you really want.

**Gonorrhea**—Sexual guilt, violation, fear. Deep feelings of shame about your sexuality. Lies. Hiding your true creativity. Too many painful relationships. Deep dislike of self. Regular self-sabotage. Holding on to dysfunctional, unhealthy relationships.

**Gout**—Experiencing too much strain, stress, and worry. Trying to control people and situations. Feeling intense pressure. Extreme stubbornness and righteousness. Seeing things only from your point of view. Feeling bound by responsibilities and principles.

**Guillain-Barré Syndrome**—Feeling attacked, criticized, weak, frozen. Inability to stand up for yourself. Feeling like your life is falling apart and you are at the lowest point. Nothing you try seems to flow. Feeling like you are just banging your head against a wall. Feeling tired of the status quo in your life and all your struggles. Wanting to give up or give in.

**Gray Hair**—Extreme stress and anxiety. Persistent worry and concern. Concentrating on old age and degeneration. Thinking, *It's all downhill from here*. Instability, shock, resistance. *See also* Baldness *and* Hair Loss.

**Growths**—Suppression, stuck emotions, frozen tears. Pushing away, rather than dealing with, problems. Hiding, covering up, burying old dreams. Feeling unfulfilled, unsatisfied, disappointed. Carrying guilt and resentment. Holding on to past failures.

# H

**Hair Loss**—Stress. Loss of protection, confidence, self-love, and direction. Feeling unattractive. Too much judgment and criticism of self and others. Frustration, guilt, resentment, anger. Pushing against the current rather than allowing things to flow in your life. *See also* Baldness *and* Gray Hair.

**Hay Fever**—Suppression of feelings. Frustration, anger, guilt, stuckness. Feeling like you can't do what you want to do. Too much worry that there is not enough (resources, finances, love, care and so on) for you to survive. No time for yourself. Needing to find out who you are allergic to, or what is irritating and infuriating you.

**Headache**—Stress, tiredness, seriousness, too much going on. Feeling out of control, overwhelmed, overcrowded, frustrated, undermined. Self-criticism, self-sabotage, invalidation of self, judgment of self and others. Too much thinking and analysis. *See also* Cluster Headache, Migraine.

**Heart Attack**—Stubbornness, stress, inflexibility, obnoxious attitude, a "my way or the highway" approach. Selfish, ignorant, controlling. Too focused on money, achievement, and winning. Neglect of your health and family. Suppression, envy, hardness. Needing to be right. Feeling unloved, easily hurt, holding on to guilt and regret. Thinking that you know everything—that you don't need anyone's help or advice.

**Heart Blockage**—Blocking love. Feeling rejected, ill-treated, inadequate, betrayed, like a failure. Difficulty accepting love and affection. Loss of hope, buried pain, stress, worry. Affecting a "don't care" attitude. Belief that you don't deserve good things in life. Feeling separate from others, cut off, lonely, isolated. Hardness toward yourself and others. Obsessed with work.

**Heartburn**—Difficulty digesting life. Guilt, anger, fear, hate. Difficulty trusting and letting go. Wanting revenge. Burning up inside. Strain. Wounded heart.

**Hemophilia**—Family-influenced belief in pain and struggle. Fragility, fear, caution, weariness. Rejection of the male side. Internal pain, degeneration.

**Hemorrhoids**—Inability to let go. A "life is unfair" attitude. Feeling guilty about or uncomfortable with past decisions. Very critical of self and others. Loss of direction and self-confidence. Anger, difficulty forgiving and learning from the past. Feeling abandoned and betrayed. Holding on to outdated family-influenced beliefs and fears.

**Hepatitis**

*All Types*—Disconnected, self-conscious, judgmental. Harsh, self-critical, stubborn, easily irritated and angered. Wanting things your own way. Finding faults with others.

Self-centered, fearful of change or transformation. Feeling resistant, guilty, ashamed, guarded.

*Type A*—Affected by other people. Judgmental. Wanting things your own way. Rebellious. Sad, anxious, frustrated, angry. Feeling like the situation you're in is unbearable. Feeling like situations keep happening over and over again. Frequent self-sabotage of your own progress.

*Type B*—Feeling powerless, disconnected from yourself, angry at the world. Feeling stuck and unable to progress or evolve to a different level. Refusing to listen to others and trying to block them out. Feeling disappointed and disillusioned by life. Numbing your feelings.

*Type C*—Self-critical, stubborn. Wanting things your own way. Easily irritated and angered. Constantly finding faults with others. Fearful, looking for someone to blame. Feeling guilty and ashamed.

*Type D*—Feeling stuck in the past. Angry that you don't know how to change the situation you are in. Trying to be who you are not, wearing a mask. Self-hatred. Fear of change and transformation. Guardedness. Self-centeredness. Acting like a victim. Looking for attention and to be saved.

**Hernia**—Abusive relationships. Controlled, taken advantage of, manipulated, exploited. Feeling stuck in a rut and that things are hopeless. Negative attitude, guilt, anger. Feeling burdened by life. Frequent self-sabotage. Blocking your creative expression.

**Herniated Disc**—Too much pressure. Not knowing when to stop. Resisting change. A need to be needed. Neglecting yourself. Difficulty asking for help. Limited thinking. Belief that there is not enough. *See also* Slipped Disk.

**Hiccups (recurring)**—Difficulty expressing your true feelings to people close to you. Confusion about decision-making. A conflict between a deep desire to please others and a need to rebel and do your own thing.

**Hip Problems**—Too much responsibility. Carrying people and problems around; a sense of burden. Too much frustration and guilt. Feeling undervalued, unacknowledged, unsupported, and unappreciated. Feeling shot down, manipulated, used, taken advantage of. Inability to move forward.

**Hives**—Profound fear, irritation, and internal explosion. Feeling overwhelmed because things are getting on top of you and you don't know how to deal with them. Deep anger and resentment. Feeling like you can't get what you want.

**Hodgkin's Disease**—Resentment, self-control, and self-punishment. Too many commitments and responsibilities. Needing to please. In a rush to achieve and receive recognition. Extreme fear of failure and of not being good enough. Holding on to toxic thoughts and beliefs.

**Huntington's Disease**—Loss of desire to move forward, to expand, and to explore. Settling for your lot in life. Loss of creativity and passion. Feeling weak, undermined. Wanting to give up or give in. Feeling like there is nothing interesting to keep you focused.

**Hyperactivity**—Scattered attention, impulsiveness, boredom, a constant need for stimulation and change. Difficulty focusing and paying attention for fear of missing out on something more interesting.

**Hypertension (high blood pressure)**—Seething inside, feeling hurt, wanting revenge. Holding on to hate, rage, and anger. Feeling too much pressure, too many demands. Wanting to be liked; trying to please others to get their attention and praise. Pushing yourself past your limit.

**Hyperthyroidism (overactive thyroid)**—Constant rushing, trying to pack as much as possible into the day. Inability to organize yourself. Under pressure and stress to achieve. Never enough time. Feeling that if you don't get things done, the world will collapse. Constant guilt about not doing more. Always there for everyone except yourself.

**Hyperventilation**—Fear, anxiety, distrust. Belief that life won't give you what you want. Resisting change. Feeling uncertain, out of control, chaotic. Too much going on. Worry, stress, strain.

**Hypoglycemia**—*See* Diabetes Types I and II.

**Hypotension (low blood pressure)**—Feeling weak, uninspired, tired. Thinking that you've had enough. Wanting to give up. Allowing others to take charge and make decisions for you. Self-neglect. Victimhood.

**Hypothyroidism (underactive thyroid)**—An "I can't be bothered" attitude. Muddled thinking, fatigue. Carrying too many burdens. Feeling worn out, emotionally unstable, exhausted. Difficulty communicating. Taking the back seat and allowing others to make important decisions. Holding back. Everything feels like too much effort.

## I

**IBS**—*See* Irritable Bowel Syndrome.

**Immune System (weak)**—Insecurity, inner conflict, self-neglect, stress. Feeling pressured, threatened, manipulated. Guard down. Allowing people to take advantage of you. Too focused on the outside world. Pushing instead of allowing.

**Impotence**—Feeling angry, pissed off, rejected. Distrust of and disconnection from your sexuality. Insecure, unsupported, fearful. Judgmental about sex. Low self-esteem. Feeling hurt by someone you loved. Fear of intimacy. Feeling vulnerable, guilty, ashamed, unlovable, depressed. Denial of joy and pleasure. Unresolved issues with your mother.

**Incontinence**—Sense of being out of control. Emotional buildup that needs releasing. Feeling anxious, timid, overwhelmed. Doubting yourself. Nagging guilt. Stress from holding on to negativity and struggle.

**Indigestion**—Difficulty assimilating experiences. Judgment, anger, unrealistic expectations. Disappointment, fear of failure. Refusal to change. Disagreements with others. Perfectionism. May be opinionated, insecure, self-righteous.

**Infection**—Feeling attacked, invaded, chaotic. Irritated, annoyed, threatened, weakened. Letting down your defenses. Feeling vulnerable. Needing attention and rest.

**Infertility**—Cold energy around the womb. Feeling rejected, abandoned, inadequate. Suppression of pain, emptiness, regret, sadness, loss, struggle, and dissatisfaction. Feeling like you are missing out on life.

**Inflammation**—Irritation, inner conflict, aggravation. Seething inside and feeling undermined. Irrational. Angry at the injustice you are seeing or experiencing. Allowing others to control and dominate you. Self-sabotage. *See also* Blepharitis (eyelid inflammation) *and* Keratitis (cornea inflammation) *under* Eye Conditions, Bone Marrow Conditions, Diverticulitis (intestinal wall inflammation), Mastitis (mammary gland inflammation), Nephritis (kidney inflammation), *and* Osteomyelitis (bone and bone marrow inflammation).

**Influenza**—Vulnerable, tired, frail. Overwhelmed by the negativity that surrounds you. Feeling like you have to carry heavy burdens that you can't handle. Feeling invalidated. Confusion and chaos inside you. In need of a "time-out." *See also* Cold (common).

**Insanity**—Inability to deal with life or to think straight. Feeling that everyone is driving you crazy. Being pushed past your boundaries. Total chaos, hopelessness, helplessness. Emotional breakdown and withdrawal. Feeling unaccepted and/or abused by your family. Needing to escape.

**Insomnia (long-term)**—Inability to relax. Feeling unsafe and unable to let go. Worrying, playing things over in your mind, dissecting situations. Feeling scattered, fearful, anxious, on guard. Harboring feelings of guilt and resentment.

**Irritable Bowel Syndrome (IBS)**—Unbalanced, too serious and controlling. Focused on the negative. Judgmental, opinionated, easily irritated. Difficulty trusting others. Holding on to outdated beliefs and ideas. Confusion, loss of direction, not knowing which way to turn.

**Itching**—Not liking what you are doing or where you are. Itching to get away. Easily irritated and annoyed. Feeling like you are getting a raw deal. Unsatisfied. Anger or resentment.

## J

**Jaundice**—Upset, irritated, bewildered, tense, furious. Feeling like you don't want to be where you are. Misunderstood, rejected, ignored. Belief that life does not support or nourish you. Resisting life. Carrying ancestral fear, apprehension, and anger.

**Jaw Problems**—Holding tension, stress, suppression. Difficulty communicating how you feel. Feeling judged, criticized, fearful. Inability to stand up for yourself and to ask for what you want. Guilt, blame, faultfinding. Feeling locked in.

**Joint Problems**—Suppressing or pushing away hurt, sadness, and frustration. Feeling lonely, unprotected, weary. Stuck in outdated beliefs. Lacking flexibility and creativity. Resistance in moving ahead. Self-righteousness.

## K

**Keratitis (inflammation of the cornea)**—*See under* Eye Conditions.

**Kidney Problems**—Low self-esteem, resentment, stuckness, exhaustion. Giving away your power, feeling unimportant. Blaming others for your shortcomings. Trying to find a scapegoat. Lack of energy. Feeling disempowered, anxious, at a loss as to what to do. A lack or breakdown of communication in relationships. Ancient sadness and fear that won't go away. *See also* Kidney Stone.

**Kidney Stone**—Hardness, negativity, inferiority. Paralyzed with fear. Wanting things your own way. Regrets, rigidity, inflexibility, stubbornness. Looking at life from a negative perspective. Living in the past. Carrying painful memories. Unable to trust. Shame, disappointment, failure. Feeling like you have been beaten up. *See also* Kidney Problems.

**Kleptomania**—Feeling depressed, ignored, and unaccepted. Needing attention. Self-loathing, guilt, shame, self-punishment. Inner conflict, unhappiness. Needing a rush.

## L

**Lactose Intolerance**—Feeling that life is difficult and that there is never enough of what you need. Resentful about your life. Wanting to be somewhere else. Belief that life is better and easier somewhere else. Lack. Needing more joy, sweetness, and creativity in your life.

**Laryngitis**—Holding back. Inability to express yourself. Can't say no. Overcommitted. Feeling guilty about something you have said or done. Internal anger and rage. Frustration; fear of criticism, rejection, and judgment. *See also* Voice (loss of).

**Leprosy**—Rejection of self. Explosive anger. Inability to handle life. Feeling unaccepted. Not belonging. Experiencing inner turmoil. Feeling unsupported, unclean, unlovable, fearful, alienated.

**Leukemia**—Lack of joy, resistance to life, self-sabotage, exhaustion, weariness. Carrying ancestral fears. Feeling that life is too hard, a struggle. Wanting to give up or be saved. Disempowerment, neglect of self and feelings. Listening to too much criticism and buying into negativity, fear, and resentment. Feeling unworthy of good things in life. *See also* Cancer.

**Lips (cracked)**—Fear of making mistakes and giving the wrong impression. Feeling bored. Sarcastic. A sense of insecurity and diminished confidence.

**Lockjaw**—Feeling strained, tainted, stuck, resistant. Unable to look after yourself or take care of things. Wanting to be somewhere else. Tension, worry, pressure. Feeling locked in, as if you have no choice.

**Lung Cancer**—Too hard on yourself and others. Too much expectation, disappointment, loneliness, bitterness, grief, heaviness, and anger. Holding on to the pain of a broken heart, or a difficult or abusive relationship. Unable to forgive and let go. Tendency to put yourself last, overdo things, and run out of energy. *See also* Cancer.

**Lupus**—Plagued by insecurity, lack of confidence, distrust. Feeling like a victim, manipulated and taken for granted. Unresolved childhood issues. Inability to stand up for yourself. Weighed down by responsibility. Always putting others first. Anger, resentment, blame, and guilt. Holding on to a belief that you need self-punishment.

**Lyme Disease**—Oversensitive. Allowing others to influence your decisions. Feeling weakened, low in energy, threatened. Too much focus on not being good enough. Beating yourself up instead of learning from your mistakes. Surrounded by critical people who constantly judge you harshly. Low self-confidence.

**Lymphoma**—Feeling threatened, anxious, afraid of loss. Toxic thoughts and outlook. Constant self-sabotage. A need to be loved, accepted, and appreciated at any cost. Always seeking people's approval by doing things for them. Hidden feelings of powerlessness, worthlessness, and insignificance. Feeling empty inside and attempting to fill that emptiness by focusing on fixing other people's problems. Making others happy instead of yourself. *See also* Cancer.

**Lymph Problems**—Feeling vulnerable, scared, unbalanced, unsupported, unloved, rejected. Easily and unfairly influenced by others. Feeling like you can't look after or protect yourself. Self-sabotage. Inability to stand up for yourself. Confusion and uncertainty. *See also* Lymphoma.

## M

**Manic Depression**—*See* Bipolar Disorder.

**Mastitis (mammary gland inflammation)**—Feeling frozen, helpless, abandoned, unsupported. Resisting change. Loss of freedom. Feeling bound by responsibilities and expectations. Pushing away your feelings. Self-neglect and self-sacrifice. Externally accommodating to others while internally fuming. Feeling left behind. Thinking life is unfair. *See also* Inflammation.

**Measles**—Feeling overwhelmed, tired, worn out, stressed, worried. Don't know how to express yourself. Inner frustration, chaos, and a sense of hopelessness. Family disharmony. In need of attention, loving care, security, and reassurance.

**Melanoma**—Feeling vulnerable and unprotected. Making limiting choices that don't work and then stubbornly sticking with them. Internal aggression that bursts to the surface. Feeling unsatisfied with life. Thinking, *Is this all there is?* Resistance to growing, changing, and expanding. Giving away your power and allowing an authority outside yourself to set the rules. Lack of trust in yourself. Refusing to research and look deeper. Wanting to be told what to do, how to think, and how to live. *See also* Cancer.

**Memory Loss**—Feeling unworthy, stressed, too focused on negativity. Caught up in life's problems. Feeling that your needs are not important. At a loss, lost, scared of the future. Thinking, *If I don't remember it, I don't have to deal with it.*

**Meningitis**—Feeling attacked, intimidated, scared. Difficulty coping with life. Experiencing inner turmoil, exhaustion, confusion, and chaos. Feeling out of balance with the flow of life and like nothing around you seems to work—as if the world has turned upside down.

**Menopausal Problems**—Fear of aging. Feeling unworthy of love and attention. Feeling sorry for yourself. Fear of not being attractive. Rejecting your feminine side. Feeling useless, past your "use by" date.

**Menstrual Problems**—Rejecting your femininity. Belief that women are weak. Constant self-criticism. Feeling disempowered, like a victim. Allowing people to push you around. Difficulty standing up for yourself. Taking life too seriously. Carrying shame and guilt about sexuality.

**Metabolic Disorders**—Difficulty assimilating information. Not knowing how to assess people accurately. Difficulty trusting. Ignoring your natural instinct. Holding on to past hurts. Easily affected by others. In some cases, harboring feelings of betrayal and disappointment.

**Migraine**—Control, pressure, seriousness, perfectionism. Overcommitting yourself. Great need for love and approval. Ignoring your own needs. Putting other people before you. Extreme guilt and anxiety. Conflict with self and other people. Self-punishment. Feeling angry and annoyed with others. Saying, "You are giving me a headache."

**Miscarriage**—Not ready for children. Fear of childbirth and responsibility. Unresolved family issues. A need of being soft, gentle, and loving with yourself. (It is possible the soul of the fetus is not ready to be born, or the body is defective and too weak to survive.)

**Morning Sickness (extreme)**—Difficulty dealing with changes in your body. Fear of being trapped. Anxiety of not being a good mother. Unresolved hurts and issues within your relationship with your partner.

**Motion Sickness**—Feeling unsafe. Unable let go and trust. Fear of being out of control.

**Mouth Ulcer (non-canker-sore form)**—Feeling stuck. Attached to destructive beliefs and points of view. Closed to new ideas. Thinking, *Life isn't fair.* Suppressing your feelings of anger and then erupting.

**Multiple Sclerosis**—Putting other people and commitments first. Pushing yourself too hard. Overworking. Not feeling good enough. Holding a limited point of view. Rejecting, neglecting, and self-sabotaging. Feeling disconnected from yourself and others. Exhaustion, worry, shame, and guilt.

**Mumps**—Difficulty swallowing other people's limiting beliefs and opinions. Not listening to your own intelligence. Feeling restrained from communicating your creative ideas. Internal conflict. Hiding what you really feel. Thinking that you are not good enough. Feeling shame related to your sexuality.

**Muscular Dystrophy**—Wasting away. Allowing, fear, grief, and sadness to eat away at you. Feeling lost, a sense of hopelessness. Taking on other people's problems and allowing these problems to trouble you. Carrying responsibilities that weigh heavily on you. Feeling that you are not important.

## N

**Nail Biting**—Nervous, unsure of yourself, unprotected. Low self-esteem. Confused, indecisive, bored, stressed. Feeling a sense of stagnation. Upset, irritated with a close family member or friend. Feeling like someone is pushing through your barriers. Nervous about an important impending event.

**Narcolepsy**—Fear of the future; avoidance, escape. Inability to cope. A sense of hopelessness and despair. Overtired. Feeling that life has become too predictable and monotonous.

**Nausea**—Fear, inability to cope with stress. Pushing problems down then needing a release. Traumatic situation that you can't watch because it makes you sick. Something that you can't handle.

**Nearsightedness**—*See under* Eye Conditions.

**Nephritis (kidney inflammation)**—Unresolved family issues, sometimes generational. Deep loneliness and longing for love and affection. Too much pressure and responsibility in everyday life. Feeling like you are drowning in your emotions and confused about what actions to take. Disappointment in either personal life or work. Too much struggle. *See also* Inflammation.

**Nervousness**—Breakdown in communication; messages not getting through. Not listening to yourself. Disconnection from yourself and others. Fear of judgment and rejection. Feeling like you need to impress or please someone. Feeling unsure of yourself and your abilities. Fear of failure. Not trusting.

**Nervous Breakdown**—Unable to handle life. Inner turmoil and confusion. People wanting too much from you. Feeling overwhelmed, strained, and hopeless. Intense anger and fear. Disappointment in self. Giving up, feeling like a failure.

**Nightmares**—Suppressed fear, stress, and anxiety manifesting through your dreams. Fears coming to the surface for you to look at and resolve. Re-emerging problems that you don't know how to deal with.

**Nodules**—Frustration, irritation, struggle. Sick of waiting for something to happen. Feeling restricted, limited, enraged. Drama.

**Nose (bleeds)**—Feeling hurt, victimized, shut out. Blaming, pointing your finger at others. Deep anger and frustration about things not happening the way you want them to. Feeling inferior, ashamed, confused. Need for attention and nourishing care.

**Nose (blocked)**—Blocking your intuition. Not listening to or resting your body. Needing time out, your own space. Feeling controlled by others. Anger that people interfere in your life and affairs.

**Nose (runny)**—Pushing, forcing, trying to make things happen instead of letting go and allowing. Ignoring your intuition and feelings. Making decisions based on reason rather than your feelings and intuition. Feeling run-down and tired of pushing, but not knowing how to stop. Propensity to interfere in other people's lives and give advice that you wouldn't take yourself. Hesitating, doubtful, not standing in your power.

**Numbness**—Suppression. Not wanting to feel, pushing your feelings down, and disconnecting from your emotions. Self-rejection. Withholding love.

## O

**Obesity**—Feeling insecure and unworthy. Needing armor to protect yourself from pain. Trying to silence feelings by overeating. Feeling unlovable. Keeping people at a distance so that they don't hurt you. Continuous self-sabotage. Conceding failure. Self-loathing and self-punishment. Stuck in a cycle of guilt, anger, and resentment. *See also* Fat *and* Overweight.

**Obsessive Compulsive Disorder (OCD)**—Inability to cope. Great need for control and predictability. Feeling unsafe, fearful, insecure, and on guard. Suspicious of things and people. Afraid that if you change, everything will go wrong and fall apart. Blaming yourself for challenging or negative events that have happened to you or to people close to you.

**Osteomyelitis (bone and bone marrow inflammation)**—Feeling deeply irritated and angered by a person or an event. Resisting confrontation. Feeling attacked, mistreated, that your trust has been broken, or that you have broken your word. Feeling isolated, worried, fearful of the future. Internal struggle related to survival and finding your place in the world. Self-sabotage. *See also* Bone Marrow Conditions *and* Inflammation.

**Osteoporosis**—Feeling weak, unsupported, limited. Holding on to guilt and resentment. Not willing to take responsibility for your actions. Self-neglect, worry. Carrying a heavy burden for others. Feeling lost, disempowered, isolated, and ashamed, as if your world is falling apart. Difficulty speaking up and asking for what you need.

**Ovarian Cancer**—Belief that women are weak and unworthy. Insecurity. Abuse survivor. Broken relationships. Deep-seated grief, terror, and anger eating at your body. Unresolved shame and humiliation. Feeling out of control and attacked, or attacking yourself. Disowning your feminine energy. Worrying, doing things for everyone else. Fear that you can't survive. *See also* Cancer.

**Ovarian Cyst**—Holding on to old hurts from men and pain from previous mental, emotional, or physical abuse. Not feeling good enough. Rejecting your femininity. Problems with fertility, like wanting a child or more children and being unable to have them. Hiding your sadness and disappointment. Feeling lonely and unloved. Conflict with your mother, sister, close female relative, or a friend. *See also* Cyst.

**Overweight**—Guilt, shame, suppressed emotions. Carrying others' problems and burdens. Trying to cover your vulnerability, hurt, or abuse from the past. Not feeling good enough. Feeling stuck. Punishing yourself with food. Trying to push people away or keep them at a distance. Not allowing your true beauty and essence to shine through. Keeping the weight as protection. Constant procrastination. *See also* Fat *and* Obesity.

## P

**Panic Attack**—Suppressed fear, anger, sadness, or painful memories that suddenly surface, often connected to past traumas, especially those from childhood. Feeling weak, stressed, undermined. Feeling attacked, criticized, pushed. Internal weakness. Overtired. Constantly resisting and going against the grain. Belief that life is full of struggle and suffering.

**Paralysis**—Unable to handle life's pressures and responsibilities. Resisting change. Stuckness. Belief that there is no choice and no way out. Feeling that nobody wants you. Rejection from family or friends. Feeling ignored or overlooked. Fear of the future. Shock stored in your body from a traumatic experience.

**Paranoia**—Fear, mistrust, obsession, blame. Suspicion that someone or something intends to hurt you. Feeling out of control. Carrying secrets that are eating at you. Thinking that something bad is going to happen.

**Parasites**—Allowing other people to feed off of your energy and life force. Feeling unclean. Infested with negativity, criticism, and frustration. Feeling like there is never enough time, energy, love, and support. Yielding to other people's demands and desires instead of your own. Giving too much without receiving enough recognition or appreciation.

**Parathyroid Problems**—Fear of failure. Disappointed in self and others. Giving up too easily. Feeling threatened by competition. Lack of belief in your ability to achieve success. Feeling controlled, especially by family members. Unsure how to break free. Feeling dependent on others. Searching for independence.

**Parkinson's Disease**—Inner conflict. Traumatic experiences that you have not dealt with. Disconnection from your feelings. No time for yourself. Feeling like a failure; useless, unlovable, unappreciated. Fear, uncertainty, inflexibility, resistance, control. Loss of hope; unfulfilled expectations, guilt. Feeling unaccepted while trying to please others. Broken spirit.

**Peptic Ulcer**—Too much worry, anxiety, and stress. Difficulty managing your time. Pushing away something that needs your urgent attention. Trying to fill the emptiness you feel with things instead of recognizing what is not working and moving forward. Anger, hurt, resentment. No outlet to express yourself. Pushing yourself too hard and too far.

**Phlegm (excessive)**—Feelings of internal and external chaos, of things spinning out of control. Difficulty saying what you really feel. Trying to be nice, suppressing your emotions. Constantly controlling yourself and how you act around others.

**Pimples (occasional)**—Frustration and angry outbursts. Not getting what you want. Feeling unaccepted and inadequate. Not liking yourself. Feeling provoked, irritated, teased. Uncomfortable in your own skin. *See also* Acne.

**Phobias**

*Aerophobia (fear of flying)*—Often occurs when you or a family member has a negative experience or accident during a flight. Also occurs from hearing or seeing visual images of plane crashes or accidents.

*Acrophobia (fear of heights, danger, death)*—Feeling weak, breakable, unbalanced, panicky. Difficulty letting go and trusting. A great need to control and have everything work. Too much thinking and visualizing worst-case scenarios. Fear of dying.

*Agoraphobia (fear of crowds and public places)*—Fear of losing control. Feeling unsupported. Difficulty trusting and asking others for help. Fear that other people will take advantage of you and hurt you. Feeling like a victim, imprisoned in your body, mind, and circumstances. Internal suffering and struggle. Feeling pent-up rage, frozen grief, helplessness, and hopelessness. Feeling that life has dealt you a cruel blow. Wanting to hide.

*Arachnophobia (fear of spiders)*—Feeling helpless, like a victim. Lack of internal power or resilience. Often connected to a childhood trauma involving spiders.

*Necrophobia (fear of death and dead things)*—Thinking, *If I avoid dead things, maybe I can escape death.* Fearing and pushing away the thought that death represents nothingness. Possibly the result of seeing someone dying or fatally ill, or having heard traumatic stories about death.

*Social Phobia (deep fear of being judged and criticized)*—A need for approval and love. Feeling left out, rejected, abandoned, and isolated. Fear of other people's anger and reactions toward you.

**PMS**—*See* Premenstrual Syndrome.

**Pneumonia**—Blocking the flow of life. Inner turmoil. Emotional hurt and anger. Exhaustion. Feeling overwhelmed and crushed by life's problems. A sense of giving up, a "What's the point? It's too hard." attitude. Desperation; drowning in your unexpressed tears and sadness. Wanting to be saved.

**Postnasal Drip**—Swallowing your anger, frustration, resentment, and sadness. Hiding how you feel inside but appearing cold, harsh, and inflexible to others. Deeply suppressed pain and aggression. Stuck in the past. Living in fantasies and dreams. Deep desire to be saved. Putting the brakes on personal expansion and evolution.

**Post-Traumatic Stress Disorder (PTSD)**—Holding on to the past. Difficulty moving forward. Stuckness, shock, guilt, regret. Feeling like a victim—threatened, hurt, weakened. Creating an internal jail, especially if you've caused trauma or death to another person. Self-punishment. Pushing people away. Fear of asking for help.

**Premature Birth**—Ignoring your own needs. Working too much. Experiencing excessive stress, violence, abuse, or trauma in your primary relationship. Feeling overwhelmed. Drinking or taking drugs. Could also be the result of irritation, vaginal infection, or fear. For the baby, impatience, discomfort, a sense of danger, a need to come out.

**Premenstrual Syndrome (PMS)**—Anger, confusion, anxiety, fear, self-doubt. Holding back ideas because you believe they will be rejected. Not being listened to. Frustrated, impatient, annoyed. Feeling trapped, unsafe, blocked, disrespected, unhappy. Holding on to past hurts from men. Feeling inferior. Denying your feminine energy. Wanting to be more masculine, to which you attribute strength and power.

**Prostate Cancer**—Struggle with work and finances. Confusion, indecisiveness. Feeling overwhelmed, undesirable, rejected, ashamed, helpless. Fear of aging. Allowing others to dictate your worth. Fear of failure. *See also* Cancer.

**Psoriasis**—Insecure, rejected, irritated. Needing to find someone to blame rather than taking responsibility. Suppressing feelings until they erupt in anger. Carrying deep disappointments. Self-hatred and self-punishment. Feeling lost, like you don't know where you belong.

**PTSD**—*See* Post-Traumatic Stress Disorder.

## R

**Rash**—Oversensitive, insecure, fearful. Self-imposed limitations that irritate or do not serve you. Small explosions of anger erupting on your skin. Feeling threatened by someone or something. Suppressed emotions that can no longer be pushed down.

**Repetitive Strain Injury (RSI)**—Not listening to your body. Difficulty letting go of the old and welcoming the new. Inflexibility, stuckness, giving away your power to someone or something else. Thinking, *I must keep doing what I don't like because I need money and can't get it any other way.* Allowing other people or situations to control you, not believing in yourself, or trusting that there is a better job or situation awaiting you. Resisting change.

**Reproductive System (problems with)**—Feeling unworthy and unlovable. Lacking confidence in yourself and your abilities. Blocking your creative expression; carrying grief about children, your childhood, family life, and past intimate relationships. Difficulty accepting yourself. Self-critical and judgmental about yourself.

**Restless Leg Syndrome (RLS)**—Uncomfortable, irritated, impatient, restless. Habitually resisting progress until you can no longer stand it and have to move forward.

Procrastinating; wanting to do something but often finding excuses not to. Frustrated that things don't happen as quickly as you want and then giving up.

**Rheumatism**—Being inflexible, domineering, superior, and self-righteous. Deep-seated resentment, anger, and bitterness. Inability to forgive and move on. Blaming others instead of taking responsibility. Belief that you are the victim of your life. Rigidity, as if everything is black or white.

**Rheumatoid Arthritis**—Self-rejection, criticism, stuckness, negativity, stubbornness. A "my way or the highway" attitude. Serious, rigid, controlling. A perfectionist; nothing ever seems good enough. Inner inflexibility, which keeps you and your joints stuck, inflamed, and in pain. Holding on to pain, sadness, regret, or guilt from the past. Refusal to change.

**Rickets**—Feeling unfulfilled and limited. Lacking adequate nourishment and support. Starving for attention, support, and help. Weakness. Struggling to take care of yourself.

**Ringworm**—Difficulty creating and keeping boundaries. Too much looking outside to ask others for advice rather than looking within. Self-sabotage. Frustration that the choices you are making don't work. Feeling limited. Desiring to be free and spontaneous but feeling bound, overpowered, and undermined. Giving your power over to someone who is freeloading off of you and your energy. *See also* Tinea.

**RLS**—*See* Restless Leg Syndrome.

**Root Canal**—Decay, deadness, self-defeating behavior, insecurity. Feeling like you are a pushover. Difficulty standing up for yourself. Swallowing other people's ideas. Feeling ashamed and inferior. Disconnecting from your roots. Rejecting an aspect of yourself.

**Rosacea**—Shame, embarrassment, guilt. Desire to be seen, acknowledged, and accepted. Overwhelmed by feelings that you have been forbidden to express. Trying to be good and to please others instead of exploring who you truly are. Constantly doubting yourself and changing your mind.

**RSI**—*See* Repetitive Strain Injury.

## S

**Scabies**—Difficulty handling life and the responsibilities that have been piled on you. Itching to get out of a situation but not knowing how. Feeling like others have the power to tell you what to do and how to do it. Lacking feelings of self-worth. Huge internal aggression and hurt. Feeling like you are being punished.

**Scarring**—Wounds that have not completely healed. A reminder of the suffering that you have experienced. Resisting change. Stuck on emotions that have not been resolved.

**Sciatica**—Feeling stuck in the past. Worried about your survival. Money issues. Unresolved feelings of inadequacy from childhood. Rejecting yourself and imposing too many limitations on yourself. Always finding excuses for why you can't do something rather than focusing on how you can. Profound fear that if you are honest, you will be neither liked nor accepted, and that you will not be able to survive. Feeling burdened with too much responsibility, which stifles your creativity.

**Scleroderma**—Feeling unattractive, unworthy, rejected, and useless. Not wanting to participate in life. Giving up or giving in. Focused on negativity, limitation, helplessness. Lack of drive or self-belief. Powerlessness and a sense of imprisonment. Feeling threatened by others, not knowing how to shield yourself from their aggression. Resisting life, which creates inflexibility of mind, body, and spirit.

**Scoliosis**—Feeling unsafe to share or reveal your true feelings. Secretive, covered up, holding back. Inability to trust others. Carrying feelings of betrayal, inferiority, low self-esteem. Feeling burdened by life. Overly responsible. Constantly criticizing self. Nothing is ever good enough. Perfectionism. Deep disappointment in life and people. Internal anger and conflict. In some cases, depression, feelings of limitation, failure, helplessness, and hopelessness.

**Seizure**—Inability to deal with life or stressful situations. Complete overload: the body needs to shut down. Having a careless attitude and denying what is occurring. Feeling overwhelmed and needing time out. Disconnection from feelings and experiences. Suppressed trauma. Withdrawal from life.

**Senility**—Loss of power and inability to deal with life; too many suppressed emotions. Regression to a childlike state, requiring constant attention from others. Overwhelmed by life, wanting to escape to another time. Not wanting to remember or to be present. Feeling lost and confused.

**Shingles**—Low self-esteem, a feeling of unworthiness that stems from childhood. Feeling slow, stupid, fearful. Holding on to anger and resentment from the past.

Fussy, demanding, hypersensitive. Constant scrutiny of self and others. Always returning to the same thought: *I'm not good enough, so I might as well give up.*

**Sickle Cell Anemia**—Feeling stuck, anxious, confused. Getting into sticky situations that are difficult to get out of. Blocking the flow of life. Making things harder than they need to be. Focus on struggle, on superficiality. Not going deep enough and discovering who you truly are. Doing things halfheartedly.

**Sinusitis**—Experiencing irritation, frustration, fear, insecurity. Trying to keep people at a distance. Repressing feelings of anger, rage, and sorrow. Carrying deep guilt and sadness from the past. Unsure how to resolve difficult situations. Overanalyzing; feeling worn out and split in too many directions. Difficulty standing up for yourself and your beliefs.

**Skin (dry)**—Feeling misunderstood. Unsure of how to express yourself and interest others in your ideas. Loss of inspiration and vitality. Feeling left out, pushed aside.

**Skin (oily)**—Out of harmony within yourself. Wanting to do more than you are doing. Rushing, pushing, making things happen. Uncomfortable in your own skin but trying to hide this feeling. Trying hard to fit in with others so that you are liked.

**Skin Cancer**—*See* Melanoma.

**Sleep Apnea**—Difficulty trusting life and letting go. Overwhelmed by problems and pressures. Repressing anger, irritation, fury. Seething inside. Trying to please others to gain their approval.

**Sleep Problems (short-term disturbances)**—Thinking too much. Unsure of how to turn off your mind. Feeling vulnerable, unprotected, unsafe, on guard. Thinking, *If I sleep and let go, someone will hurt me or take advantage of me.* Extreme fear and anxiety. Feeling threatened and helpless. Unresolved problems.

**Sleep Walking**—Energies that you can no longer repress when you sleep. Feeling out of control. Fear of showing people who you really are. Thinking that something bad or dark is inside you, and that people will reject, ridicule, and abandon you if they discover it. The need to explore yourself and allow your spontaneity to surface.

**Slipped Disc**—Difficulty making decisions. Feeling emotionally unsupported. Lack of trust; emotional blockages holding you back. Neglecting your needs. Too much pressure, creating stiffness and immobility in your body. *See also* Herniated Disk.

**Smell (loss of)**—Ignoring your intuition. Feeling stuck. Surrounded by toxic people and energy. Lack of creativity and spontaneity. Trying to control yourself too much around others. Perfectionism.

**Snoring**—Not wanting to let go of old ways of thinking or doing things. A need to control. Feeling like you can't express what you need to say. Fear of change.

**Social Anxiety**—*See* Social Phobia *under* Phobias.

**Sore Throat**—Not saying what you really feel. Holding yourself back. Feeling stressed, frustrated, angry, fearful. Internal conflict. Fear of not being accepted. *See also* Strep Throat.

**Spasms**—Feeling stressed, anxious, tense, resistant, frustrated. Apprehensive about the future.

**Spastic Colitis**—Stress, anxiety, worry. Feeling contracted inside. Usure of how to deal with an issue. Focused on problems rather than solutions. Lack of trust. Constantly changing your mind and second-guessing your instinct. Feeling attacked and criticized by others. On guard because you don't want to get hurt.

**Spinal Curvature**—*See* Scoliosis.

**Sprain**—Feeling scattered, unfocused, vague. Needing to pay attention. Pushing past your limits. Impatient, intolerant. Irritated with someone or something. Oblivious to what is going on. Making silly mistakes and regularly misjudging things. Resisting authority.

**Stiff Neck**—Problems with people. Feeling stuck in a limited point of view. Difficulty making commitments. Feeling pressured, like someone is pressing on you—pushing you to do what you don't want to do. Thinking too much. Trying to dissect rather than feel.

**Stiffness**—Limitation, stuckness, fear. Being indecisive, controlling, a perfectionist. A "my way or the highway" attitude. Acting self-righteous, giving off a superior attitude, believing that you are all-knowing. Inability to handle challenges or mistakes constructively and positively.

**Stomach Ulcer**—*See* Ulcer (stomach).

**Strep Throat**—Anger, rage, hurt, hatred, stubbornness. Feeling inferior. Don't know how to say no or to stand up for yourself, even though you are burning inside. listening to yourself and your own guidance. Fearful of the future and how you will survive. *See also* Sore Throat.

**Stretch Marks**—Feeling stretched to the limit. Don't know how you will cope with the future. Feeling uncomfortable in your skin. Judging yourself and your body harshly. Resistant to change.

**Stroke**—Feeling useless, hopeless, inadequate. Overwhelming pressure and stress. Unable to handle the situation you are in. Giving up. Feeling like a failure. Shutting down. Refusing to change and failing to understand why what you have done did not work.

**Sty**—*See under* Eye Conditions.

**Sun Stroke**—Don't know when to stop. Pushing the boundaries and limits of what is possible. Belief that the usual rules don't apply to you. Rebellion. Self-neglect.

**Surgery (slow recovery)**—Feeling helpless, guilty, frustrated, unsupported. Needing more love and attention. Not honoring your body or giving it enough rest. Feeling stuck and hardened. Not trusting that your body knows how to heal.

**Stuttering**—Feeling insecure, inadequate, self-conscious, limited, boxed in. Difficulty communicating with others. Holding back and not sharing how you feel. Suppressing your creativity. Buying into other people's criticisms and limiting ideas about yourself and your abilities.

**Swelling**—Carrying negative beliefs and feelings that fester in your body and block your health and success. Suppressing old grief and pain, allowing it to grow until your body swells. Carrying frozen tears that need to melt and come out.

**Syphilis**—Feeling threatened, powerless, victimized, vulnerable, intimidated, invisible, unimportant, unworthy, unwanted. Neither listened to nor heard. Carrying shame, guilt, resentment, anger. Unsure of how or when to say no and how to create healthy boundaries. Allowing others to use and discard you. Self-sabotage, self-rejection, and self-loathing.

# T

**Tapeworm**—Living off someone, or allowing someone to use you and your resources. Feeling like people are sucking your life force away and controlling you. Thinking, *How do I get hooked into others' problems and drama?* An urgent need to take back your power and redirect your life.

**Teeth Grinding**—Unable to let go of or deal with everyday stresses. Holding on to anger or fear from the past. Worry about the future. Inability to make up your mind, or to relax and unwind. Feeling that you have too much to deal with, too many decisions to make. Biting off more than you can chew.

**Thrombosis**—Stuckness. Not allowing yourself to follow your heart. Resisting life; pushing, limiting, procrastinating. Disconnected from your internal wisdom. Holding in anger and resentment. Feeling threatened. Focused on difficulty, struggle, and challenges.

**Thrush**—*See* Candida.

**Tics/Twitches**—Stress, apprehension, anxiety, excitement. Unsure of how to react to a situation. Shock. Fear of the future. *See also* Tourette's Syndrome.

**Tinea**—Allowing old beliefs that do not serve you to fester under your skin and feed off of you. Holding on to old anger and disappointment. Feeling irritated and frustrated because you aren't getting what you want. Impatience, edginess, intolerance, arrogance, pride, and superior attitude, none of which allow you to change. *See also* Ringworm.

**Tinnitus**—Too much going on in your life, shutting down your ability to hear or listen. Not trusting your own inner guidance. Stubborn.

**Tonsillitis**—Feeling defensive, controlling, fearful. Believing that what you have to express is not important and that others will not want to hear it. Suppressing your creativity and joy. Underestimating your talents and abilities. Clinginess. Seeking others' permission and support for what you do.

**Tourette's Syndrome**—Feeling out of control, suppressed, frustrated, confused, afraid to speak. Misunderstood by others. Ancient hurt. Victimized. Sad, lonely, depressed. Distrust of self and your body. Afraid that there is something dark or bad inside you. Pushing things away or aside until you can no longer handle them and explode. *See also* Tics/Twitches.

**Tuberculosis**—Feeling weak, inferior, overpowered, angry. Inner turmoil and struggle. Afraid that others want to take advantage of and defeat you. Trying to protect yourself by hurting others first. In some cases, selfishness, and possessive traits and behaviors.

**Trauma (emotional)**—Feeling fragile, weak, and lost, like the world has caved in. Betrayal, disappointment. Lack of care and support. Stuck, frozen, cold. Disconnected from your guidance and higher purpose.

**Trauma (physical)**—Not listening to your own or to Universal Guidance. Deeply resisting change. Needing a wake-up call. Constantly limiting yourself by allowing negative thinking to take over your life. Self-sabotage.

**Tumors**—Shock, fear, trauma, self-neglect, not following through with promises. Breaking agreements with yourself and others. Suppressing emotional hurt. Feelings of anger, revenge, and resentment. Difficulty in believing and trusting others. Feeling unlovable. Believing that nobody cares about you. Experiencing jealousy and envy toward others.

## U

**Ulcer (gastrointestinal)**—Holding on to anger, fear, hatred, rage, disappointment, grief, bitterness, sorrow. Excessive worry, not trusting in life. On guard, controlling. Perfectionism. Feeling helpless, powerless, and unworthy. Carrying overwhelming responsibility. Resenting having to do things for other people, especially when they do not appreciate you. Self-sabotage, self-inflicted pain; wanting revenge or payback.

**Ulcer (stomach)**—Negative outlook. Feeling like nothing or nobody makes you happy. Not knowing what you want or how to take care of yourself. Feeling lost, alone, isolated, abandoned, rejected. Difficulty knowing how to receive love, help, or abundance. Too much worry and anxiety. Fear of the future and of change.

**Underweight**—Lacking nourishing, loving attention. Taking things out on yourself; punishing yourself. Guilt, criticism, unhappiness, disapproval. Holding yourself back from expansion and growth.

**Urethritis**—Feeling vulnerable, attacked, shot down, like a failure. Acting against your beliefs. Feeling that life is unfair and that you are a victim of your circumstances. Holding on to unresolved sadness and grief from the past.

**Urinary Tract Infection (UTI)**—Seeking someone to blame for your problems or shortcomings. Feeling pissed off, irritated, angry, bitter. Carrying a tremendous amount of guilt and fear. A deep-seated belief that there is something wrong with you.

Allowing people to manipulate and control you. Not knowing how to stand up for yourself and say no. Sexual pressure and shame.

**UTI**—*See* Urinary Tract Infection.

# V

**Vaginitis**—Shame and guilt about your sexuality. Feeling victimized, wounded by past relationships, disgraced, humiliated, embarrassed. Feeling you've done something wrong or that someone has wronged you, and unable to forgive and move on. Degrading yourself. Blame and anger toward others.

**Varicose Veins**—Difficulty receiving love. Blocking your ability to move forward. Feeling stuck, fearful, helpless, unsupported. A sense of being trapped without seeing a way out. Belief that nothing works for you; no matter what you try, nothing changes. Feeling like you are living a lie and not tapping into your full potential. Too much pressure, stress, and responsibility. Carrying such a big load that your legs can no longer support you. Disappointed, especially about your employment.

**Venereal Disease**—Feeling seduced, out of control, ashamed, humiliated. Wanting to run away and hide. Feeling guilty, like you have done something sinful. Experiencing rejection, fear, or an invalidation of self. Angry with yourself or your partner.

**Vertigo**—The body in overload. Feeling unstable, out of balance, ungrounded, confused. Unable to handle life. Things seeming different than you'd thought them to be. Feeling unsafe, scattered, burdened. Wanting to hide or to be somewhere else. Difficulty accepting things as they are. Going round and round in circles but not sure how to make changes, or which direction to take.

**Viruses**—Feeling out of control, vulnerable, easily manipulated and affected by others, criticized, harassed, threatened, attacked, like a victim.

**Voice (loss of)**—Experiencing a sense of powerlessness, hopelessness, and stuckness. Pushing yourself beyond your capacity. Refusing to listen to your inner guidance and communicate your feelings to others. Feeling like you have lost your voice, your power. Confused. Conflicted about your feelings. *See also* Laryngitis.

**Vomiting**—Carrying more heaviness, stress, and stuckness than your body can take.

## W

**Warts**—Viewing life as ugly, threatening, hostile. Focusing on negativity, and what you hate and dislike, rather than on what you like or love. Feeling inadequate, unattractive, unworthy of good things in life.

**Water Retention**—Holding on to heavy or limiting emotions from the past. Difficulty moving forward. Swimming in sadness and hopelessness. Not knowing how to live your life in happiness. Constant self-sabotage. Resisting your feelings rather than learning from them. Pushing away from what you want. Family conflicts.

**Whiplash**—A jolt to indicate that you need to make changes in your life. Confusion, self-criticism, and attack. Beating yourself up or allowing others to prey on you.

**Whooping Cough**—Pushing people away. Feeling like you need your own space and distance. Feeling completely overwhelmed, scared, and stressed. Deep internal rage. Experiencing a sense of powerlessness. Lack of freedom to express yourself. Feeling misunderstood, taken for granted, criticized, taken advantage of.

**Worms (parasites)**—Allowing other people to feed off you. Feeling overwhelmed, undervalued, rejected. Thinking that you are dirty and that there is something wrong with you. Discomfort with your body. Feeling like everyone wants a piece of you.

**Wounds**—Suppressed hurts that come to the surface of your body as wounds. Feeling like a victim. Self-criticism and judgment. Difficulty forgiving.

# III

# THE SECRET LANGUAGE OF YOUR EMOTIONS

## Understanding and Healing Emotions That Cause Disease

In this section, you will find a brief explanation of how emotions can affect health and impact our life experience by contributing to various diseases and ailments.

Many of us suppress our unpleasant emotions unconsciously as a protective mechanism because, on some level, we believe that we cannot handle pain or the multitude of other possible feelings. I have found in my clients' experiences and my own life that emotions do not disappear simply because we don't allow ourselves to feel them or we suppress them. In fact, emotions often stay in the body until they are recognized, acknowledged, and released. If this process does not happen, dense and heavy emotions can contribute to disease and disfunction.

I have worked with many people who have discovered stagnant emotions from thirty, forty, and fifty years ago (or longer), that caused them difficulty, unhappiness, and ill health until they were able to release them.

Take Lauren's inspiring story, for example. She came to see me when she was sixty-five years old, having been depressed since she was ten. Lauren felt that to be accepted she had to please everyone, and she did not know how to say no. After recognizing the load she carried, she regularly began to practice some of the emotional clearing processes described in this book. Within a short time, Lauren was almost unrecognizable. She stood tall, felt empowered, and spoke confidently, as though what she had to say really mattered. She began to say no to others when appropriate and yes to herself. And most of all, she enjoyed being Lauren.

Following Lauren's dramatic transformation, people began to comment on how good she looked, how happy she seemed, and how much they enjoyed spending time with her. She began to work with younger people, inspiring them to do their best. Finally connected to her authentic self, Lauren let go of the limitations she had placed on herself about what she could do or be, and started living the fulfilling, inspiring life she had always desired.

Another client, Tess, suffered from frequent headaches for many years. When she was younger, her mother had been very judgmental, and Tess learned to be self-critical, insecure, and controlling. When Tess recognized those traits in herself, she began to use the processes to clear them, and within a few weeks, her headaches stopped. Tess worked on many aspects of herself in order to feel more emotionally balanced. She even taught her young children to express their emotions in a healing way, with positive results for their own ailments.

When I started working with Jason, he was overweight and had severe backache and stomach cramps. He had worked in a corporate environment for seventeen years and had recently divorced. Jason carried a lot of guilt and resentment in his body about his family's breakup. He realized that, in order to move forward and reestablish a healthy relationship with his ex-wife and children, he needed to release his anger, resentment, and guilt and allow more peace and forgiveness into his life. As Jason shed his resentment and guilt, he also shed thirty-three pounds. His backache and stomach cramps disappeared, and he became more sensitive to his own needs and the needs of others. His children also benefited, as he began to spend quality time with them, teaching them to listen to and express their feelings.

As my clients' experiences suggest, using these clearing processes will often have a tremendous impact on your family, friends, and all those you are in contact with as well. How often have you gone somewhere feeling tense or stressed and then met someone who inspired you to change, or who made you feel wonderful? In the past, you may have felt that you didn't have a choice because you did not know how to change, but now the tools are at your fingertips. I hope that these stories of success will inspire you to take action and use these processes to transform your own life. I believe that, given the right tools, we all have the capacity to experience peace, clarity, and joy. I have worked with thousands of people who have changed their lives using these simple processes. I would love for you to be one of those people.

As it would have been too much to include all the challenging emotions in one book, I wanted to provide you with a general process, which you can apply to any emotion you would like to release. To assist you even further, I have created a free audio download to help you release stuck emotions, which can be accessed on my website. The link is listed at the back of this book.

## Process to Identify and Release Unhealthy Emotions

The majority of part III is about healing yourself by releasing dense, unhealthy emotions, but before you can release these emotions, you must identify them. While I may refer to positive and negative energy in relation to emotions, it is important to understand that emotions are not unhealthy or negative in themselves. All emotions are important and contain blessings. So, for the purposes of your work here, it makes more sense to refer to healthy and unhealthy emotions, in the sense that if you hold on to them or get stuck with them for long periods of time, they will affect your health and lead to illness. Each emotion contains a lesson or a gift, and it is for you to find it. In order to do this process, find a quiet, comfortable place and, with a pen and paper handy, do the following:

1. Connect to your emotions. You can do this by focusing your attention within and noticing which parts of your body heavy emotions are being stored in.

2. When you are aware of the affected part or parts of the body, place your hands there and breathe deeply into the emotion for a minute or two. As you breathe, ask if this feeling has any messages for you.

3. Listen for the response. You may hear a word that gives you an insight into something you have been experiencing over and over again, or you may remember a challenging experience in your life that you have not expressed or healed. Whatever your experience, do not judge it.

4. Write down any insights you receive, and explore their significance. Complete the clearing process described in each section until you can feel that the density and negativity of those emotions have been released from your body and replaced by your expanded consciousness, light, and peace.

5. When you have cleared the negativity from the emotion, complete the corresponding positive aspect listed at the end of each clearing process. This will help you finish transforming the energy in your body from negative to positive. Furthermore, the processes involving positive emotions, such as confidence, joy, and peace, may also be used on their own to help you foster those feelings within yourself.

## *Releasing Unhealthy Emotions*

Once you have identified an unhealthy emotion, look for the corresponding section offered and perform the process to release this emotion. When you say the words in the processes, allow yourself to really feel what you are saying. Say the words out loud so that you can feel the magnitude of their power. If it is not possible to say them out loud, focus on how each word affects you as you read it or say it quietly to yourself.

Similarly, visualize or sense the orange-red color moving through your body, cleansing it. I recommend using orange light to help clear dense or heavy emotions, as this hue has the ability to bring emotions to the surface for healing and transformation. It is also a color that stimulates movement, energy, warmth, and enthusiasm.

In my "The Secret Language of Your Emotions" workshops, I have discovered that music can be highly beneficial in releasing many of the challenging feelings people experience. For example, if you are feeling angry or frustrated, shaking your body vigorously to loud music may help free the charge, making the release exercise more effective. If you are stuck, then soft, fluid movements to flowing music may help as you allow your mind to find new ways of seeing the challenge or the situation you are stuck in. To release control, staccato movements while imagining yourself breaking the chains of control may help. In other words, be creative by combining breath, movement, feelings, touch, and visualization together.

If you are having trouble releasing particularly difficult emotions, I have also created audio programs which can further assist you, described at the back of this book.

## Anger

Anger often comes out of righteousness, fear, or judgment that arises when people feel they have been wronged or haven't gotten what they want. Rather than taking responsibility, they blame others. Anger gives people a false sense of power, making them feel justified to criticize, put down, hate, and resent others. Angry people feel the right to fight, to hurt someone, or to treat people badly.

On the other hand, anger can be a catalyst for change and transformation by fueling your passion, excitement, and enthusiasm. If something in your life is not working and you are angry, this anger offers an opportunity for you to free yourself from your ailment, such as depression, powerlessness, feeling overwhelmed, and so on. However, if protracted, anger drains energy and life force. Long-term anger can leave a person feeling fatigued, frail, unhappy, and worn out.

Unresolved anger contributes to hypertension, inflammation, psoriasis, sinusitis, tumors, cancers, premenstrual syndrome, pneumonia, tinea, ulcers, and more.

### Process to Release Anger:

• Place your hands on the part of your body where you feel anger most intensely. Breathe into the area for a few moments, allowing any emotion to rise to the surface with little resistance.

• Relax your hands.

• Say: "Divine Healing Intelligence, pour the orange-red flame of purification into every aspect of my being that is holding on to anger, hatred, hurt, and thoughts of revenge. Please dissolve all feelings of fear, numbness, rage, and judgment. Allow me to find new healing ways to express and let go of anger. Help me to realize that anger is not who I am; it is an emotion I have bought into and have been afraid to release. But now I am ready for something better, softer, and healthier. I am willing to transform anger into peace. Thank you."

• Repeat the word "CLEAR" several times until you feel lighter.

• Observe the orange-red flame moving through your body, mind, emotions, and energy field, and begin to dissolve all negative thoughts, words, feelings, memories, and images of anger, rage, superiority, judgment, numbness, and fear.

• Bring back feelings of peace and tranquility using the Peace process on page 204.

## Anxiety—*See* Fear.

## Attack—*See* Criticism.

## Control

Many people limit themselves and their opportunities by trying to control themselves and the people around them, creating a lot of stress, worry, and tension. The need for control arises from people feeling that their lives cannot be perfect unless they dictate and dominate other people's actions. They believe they need to create a multitude of rules to "order" their lives and the lives of others. Need for control and perfectionism imply a lack of trust and belief in yourself and others. It keeps people limited and disconnected from their hearts.

Control often becomes aggression when the person or experience someone is trying to control does not comply. Controlling types fear spontaneity, creativity, imagination, and fun because these things break down oppression, constriction, and restriction.

On a physical level, control can bring about brain tumors, acne, agoraphobia, allergies, anorexia, asthma, baldness, bulimia, cancer, deafness, diabetes, frozen shoulder, frigidity, gout, hernia, Hodgkin's disease, inflammation, irritable bowel syndrome, migraines, ovarian cancer, paranoia, Parkinson's disease, repetitive-strain injuries, headaches, and ulcers, among other problems.

**Process to Release Control:**

• Place your hands on the part of your body where you feel control most intensely. Breathe into the area for a few moments while allowing any emotion to rise to the surface with little resistance.

• Then relax your hands.

• Say: "Divine Healing Intelligence, using the orange-red flame of light, please dissolve my need to control, manipulate, and dominate. Help me release the stress of keeping rules and wanting things my own way. Free me from controlling others or being controlled. Help me become more flexible, expansive, spontaneous, and open-minded. Thank you."

• Repeat the word "CLEAR" several times until you feel lighter.

• Observe the orange-red flame of light moving through your body, mind, emotions, and energy field, and begin to clear and dissolve all negative thoughts, words, feelings, memories, and images of control and manipulation. Allow yourself to experience the freedom of choice, creativity, and spontaneity.

• In order to bring back feelings of freedom and choice, do the Freedom process on page 201.

## Criticism

Whenever you become self-critical, self-deprecating, or take on other people's criticisms of you, your body begins to lose its life force and weaken. Your bones and muscles find it difficult to support the weight of criticism and negativity, and they deteriorate.

Fear of criticism, just like fear of failure, can stop you from following your heart, which can make life less interesting and fun. Being criticized and attacked over long periods often leads to low self-esteem and self-worth, and can cause depression.

Whether people are criticizing or accepting others' criticisms, they are placing energetic knives into themselves that limit and hold them back from their power. The expression "backstabbing" refers to the act of criticizing someone. Long-term criticism can lead to a nervous system disorder, heart attack, hemorrhoids, liver problems, or hepatitis.

**Process to Release Criticism:**
• Place your hands on the part of your body where you feel attacked and criticized most intensely. Breathe into the area for a few moments, allowing any emotion to rise to the surface with little resistance.

• Relax your hands.

• Say: "Divine Healing Intelligence, using the orange-red flame of purification, please dissolve all thoughts, feelings, and experiences of attack, criticism, weakness, irritation, and anger from my body and consciousness. Dissolve all energetic attacks and knives in my back. Help me release blame, shame, limitation, and all the negative programming I have picked up from other people. Awaken courage, compassion, and a belief in myself. Thank you."

• Repeat the word "CLEAR" several times until you feel lighter.

• Observe the orange-red flame moving through your body, mind, emotions, and energy field, and begin to dissolve all negative thoughts, words, feelings, memories, and images of criticism, attack, negative programming, weakness, and limitation.

• To bring back feelings of praise and encouragement, do the Encouragement process on page 199.

## Depression

Depression has become a monumental problem for many people who are overwhelmed by the pressure to make ends meet and survive in our increasingly complex society.

Hopelessness and depression can arise from deep disappointment, betrayal, the loss of a loved one, failure, anger turned inward, an accident, a major trauma, or a physiological condition. Depression can make you feel helpless, misguided, confused, fatigued, and melancholy. You may feel that life has lost its meaning, and has become dull, colorless, and pointless. You may experience being trapped in the darkness of your mind and find it difficult to see a way out.

However, depression can also provide you with the opportunity to connect to and work with the aspects within yourself that you have not accepted and have repressed. Working with these aspects can not only lead to a deeper understanding of yourself, but profound healing and transformation as well.

Physically, depression can lead to problems with the chest, lungs, blood, gallbladder, gallstones, and prostate, as well as back pain, alcoholism, compulsive eating, scoliosis, joint stiffness, abscess, Alzheimer's disease, amnesia, and many other ailments.

**Process to Release Depression:**
• Place your hands on the part of your body where you feel your depression most intensely. Breathe into the area for a few moments, allowing any emotion to rise to the surface with little resistance.

• Relax your hands.

• Say: "Divine Healing Intelligence, using the orange-red ray of light, sweep away all depression, disappointment, dullness, and helplessness from my system. Help me find my way out of this heavy, dreary state and renew my life force, so that I can begin to see the brighter side of life, full of joy, laughter, and fun. Restore my enthusiasm and thirst for life so that I can contribute to humanity, and give back all the kindness and assistance I have been blessed to receive. Thank you."

• Repeat the word "CLEAR" several times until you feel lighter.

• Observe the orange-red ray of light moving through your body, mind, emotions, and energy field, and begin to clear and dissolve all negative thoughts, words, feelings, memories, and images of depression and disappointment.

- Bring back feelings of joy and vivacity using the Joy process on page 203.

## Discrimination—*See* Judgment.

## Envy—*See* Jealousy.

## Failure

Many people evaluate themselves and their endeavors as failures, using this label as an excuse to stop pursuing their goals. Or they may use fear of failure as an excuse, believing that their dream is too hard or impossible to achieve. When people feel they have failed, they experience disappointment and letdown, which then causes depression and hopelessness.

The positive effect of failure is the opportunity to discover a different way of achieving what we want. It can inspire us to become creative and to look at past failures as stepping stones toward achieving great success. We can reflect on what we have learned from difficult situations and move forward with greater confidence and belief in ourselves.

On a physical level, failure may contribute to farsightedness, gallstones, nervous breakdown, scoliosis, cold sores, stroke, prostate cancer, back pain, blood pressure, compulsive eating, conjunctivitis, cysts, fibroid tumors, frozen shoulder, heart blockage, Hodgkin's disease, indigestion, kidney stones, obesity, and Parkinson's disease, among other conditions.

### Process to Release Feelings of Failure:
- Place your hands on the part of your body where you feel failure and disappointment most intensely. Breathe into the area for a few moments, allowing any emotion to rise to the surface with little resistance.

- Relax your hands.

- Say: "Divine Healing Intelligence, using the orange-red sword of light, please cut me loose from all the fear, worry, and anxiety about failing to achieve my goals. Release and dissolve all disappointment and frustration about past letdowns and setbacks. Allow me to charge forward with a renewed belief in myself, and in my abilities to succeed and accomplish wonderful things, contributing to my life and to other people's lives. Help me to become aware that my failures can be turned into successes. Remind me to appreciate all the success I already have in my life, and open the doors for more. Thank you."

• Repeat the word "CLEAR" several times until you feel lighter.

• Observe the orange-red light of the sword moving through your body, mind, emotions, and energy field, and begin to cut and dissolve all negative thoughts, words, feelings, memories, and images of failure, disappointment, and frustration.

• In order to bring back feelings of success and fulfillment, do the Success process on page 207.

## Fear

People fear the future based on their past experiences. Fearful people are capable of betrayal, lies, prejudice, treachery, blame, rejection, harm, and violence. Fear locks a person into negativity, creating shock, anxiety, stress, and worry. It can also inhibit change and progress, as many people feel comfortable with what they know and fear of change makes them stuck where they are, afraid to move forward. Fear controls, paralyzes, and imprisons. It prevents people from taking action, trusting themselves, and achieving their goals. It sabotages people's efforts by constantly creating setbacks, so that they feel powerless. Fear also creates a sense of separation and vulnerability, and concern that someone else has power over us. Fear impairs judgment, clouds thinking, and limits—even blocks—our ability to love, and experience peace and joy.

Fear contributes to many health conditions, including ulcers, urinary tract infections, venereal diseases, tumors, cancers, insomnia, sinusitis, sciatica, back pain, Parkinson's disease, obsessive-compulsive disorder, impotence, hepatitis, hemorrhoids, diabetes, cysts, anorexia, and agoraphobia.

**Process to Release Fear:**

• Place your hands on the part of your body where you feel fear most intensely. Breathe into this area for a few moments while allowing any emotion to rise to the surface with little resistance.

• Relax your hands.

• Say: "Divine Healing Intelligence, using the orange-red flame of purification, please dissolve all fear, anxiety, worry, and powerlessness. Help me release feelings of helplessness, hopelessness, betrayal, and trauma. Help me to find a blessing in every challenging situation and to focus on the best possible outcome. Thank you."

• Repeat the word "CLEAR" several times until you feel lighter.

• Observe the orange-red flame moving through your body, mind, emotions, and energy field, and begin to dissolve all negative thoughts, words, feelings, memories, and images of fear, anxiety, worry, and powerlessness.

• To bring back feelings of love and empowerment, do the Love process on page 203.

## Feeling Overwhelmed

In this modern age, people are easily overwhelmed by the amount of information and choices available. This overload of information can often lead to confusion, uncertainty, and a sense of chaos.

The load of responsibility that many people carry is increasingly bigger and heavier; there is always too much to do and not enough time or resources to do it. The pressure of trying to do too much can become overwhelming and lead to stress, fatigue, and exhaustion.

Physically, feeling overwhelmed contributes to back pain, breast issues, headaches, shoulder and ankle problems, Alzheimer's disease, blackouts, colds, deafness, glaucoma, nervous breakdown, prostate cancer, seizure, senility, stroke, and ulcers.

**Process to Release Overwhelming Feelings:**

• Place your hands on the part of your body where you feel most intensely overwhelmed. Breathe into the area for a few moments while allowing any emotion to rise to the surface with little resistance.

• Relax your hands.

• Say: "Divine Healing Intelligence, using the orange-red flame of light, please sweep through my entire system, clearing all stress, fatigue, and overwhelming feelings. Please help me to let go of the heavy burdens I carry and allow me to see a lighter, more balanced side of life. Help me turn chaos into order, uncertainty into self-belief, and confusion into clarity. Allow me to find equilibrium in my life so that I can embrace and enjoy each step of my life's journey. Thank you."

• Repeat the word "CLEAR" several times until you feel lighter.

• Observe the orange-red light moving through your body, mind, emotions, and energy field, and begin to clear and dissolve all negative thoughts, words, overwhelming feelings, memories, and images of confusion and chaos.

• In order to bring back feelings of balance and clarity, do the Clarity process on page 197.

## Frustration

Frustration is one of the most common emotions. It has an element of impatience, struggle, suffering, and irritation. Often, people become frustrated when things aren't flowing their way, when they feel a situation should be different than it is, or when they have to wait for something to happen. Long-term frustration becomes aggression, irritation, inflammation, and attack.

In its positive role, frustration may be the driving force you need to change the way you are living your life.

Physically, frustration can contribute to problems with the eyes, feet (including athlete's foot), gallbladder, large intestine, sinuses, skin conditions, nodules, celiac disease, and sleep apnea.

**Process to Release Frustration and Irritation:**
• Place your hands on the part of your body where you feel frustration or irritation most intensely. Breathe into the area for a few moments while allowing any emotion to rise to the surface with little resistance.

• Relax your hands.

• Say: "Divine Healing Intelligence, using the orange-red flame of light, please move through every part of my body and mind, dissolving all feelings, thoughts, and patterns of frustration, irritation, and aggravation. Please sweep away all impatience, struggle, and suffering that resides in my consciousness. Allow me to turn my frustration into inspiration and enthusiastic action. Help to steer me in the direction where my actions will become actualized so that I can experience satisfaction with my accomplishments. Thank you."

• Repeat the word "CLEAR" several times until you feel lighter.

• Observe the orange-red light moving through your body, mind, emotions, and energy field, and begin to clear and dissolve all negative thoughts, words, feelings, memories, and images of frustration, irritation, and aggravation.

• Bring back feelings of satisfaction and inspiration by doing the Satisfaction process on page 206.

## Grief
People often feel sad when they feel that they have lost something. Although grief is an important part of healing, when suppressed, it can lead to depression, victimhood, self-pity, hopelessness, blame, unhappiness, and sickness.

Many experience sadness from the loss of a loved one, a job, an opportunity, their youth, or a marital breakdown. Moving to a different country and leaving loved ones may similarly cause grief from feelings of not belonging, isolation, and loss of identity.

Sadness and grief must be recognized and expressed in order to heal; loss can be extremely difficult. Each person deals with loss differently, and though the time it takes to heal may vary, prolonged sadness and grief can keep you focused on the past, and limit you from moving forward.

Sadness, grief, and loss can lead to sinusitis, pneumonia, frozen shoulders, kidney problems, ovarian cysts, muscular dystrophy, Parkinson's disease, memory loss, lower back pain, carpal tunnel syndrome, irritable bowel syndrome, hemorrhoids, heart problems, anemia, and many other conditions.

**Process to Release Sadness:**

• Place your hands on the part of your body where you feel sadness most intensely. Breathe into the area for a few moments while allowing any emotion to rise to the surface with little resistance.

• Relax your hands.

• Say: "Divine Healing Intelligence, using the orange-red flame of purification, please help me heal all sadness, grief, and loss. Help me release all blame, self-pity, confusion, and unhappiness I am carrying. Please dissolve the intense ache, longing, and depression I am feeling. Allow me to gain insights into the hidden blessings of my sadness and grief, and to grow wiser and stronger. Thank you."

• Repeat the word "CLEAR" several times until you feel lighter.

• Observe the orange-red light moving through your body, mind, emotions, and energy field, and begin to clear and dissolve all negative thoughts, words, feelings, memories and images of sadness, grief, blame, and self-pity.

• To bring back feelings of happiness, do the Happiness process on page 201.

## Guilt

The whole justice system is based on the guilty and the innocent, and we all know that guilt has strong consequences. Consciously or subconsciously, guilt is associated with punishment, jail, and the need to serve a sentence. Guilt also requires judgment, which can lead to shame and embarrassment. Guilt and shame eat away at the body because many people hold the self-sabotaging belief that they deserve to be punished.

People feel guilty about working too much, not working enough, not spending enough time with their kids, spending too much money, drinking too much, and so on. Even relaxation, rest, or having more money or luxuries than others can lead to guilt. In addition, guilt often encourages people to do the very thing they feel guilty about. An easy example is eating sweets or junk food: the guiltier someone feels about them, the more they are likely to eat them.

All guilt is the same; it is destructive to your body and soul. It keeps you in chains rather than helping you change and discover freedom.

Guilt is associated with hip problems, migraines, weight issues, venereal disease, osteoporosis, Parkinson's disease, insomnia, sinusitis, impotence, hernia, and heart disease.

### Process to Release Guilt:

• Place your hands on the part of your body where you feel guilt most intensely. Breathe into the area for a few moments while allowing any emotion to rise to the surface with little resistance.

• Relax your hands.

• Say: "Divine Healing Intelligence, using the orange-red flame of purification, please dissolve all thoughts, feelings, and memories of guilt, regret, and judgment from my consciousness. Help me let go of self-punishment, limitation, and self-sabotage. Work with me to release patterns of shame, embarrassment, and destruction. I am now willing to let go of all the heavy burdens that are weighing me down so that I can be free. Thank you."

• Repeat the word "CLEAR" several times until you feel lighter.

• Observe the orange-red flame moving through your body, mind, emotions, and energy field, and begin to dissolve all negative thoughts, words, feelings, memories, and images of guilt, self-punishment, judgment, and regret.

• In order to bring back the feeling of innocence and purity, do the Innocence process on page 202.

## Hatred

Hatred shows itself in many ways, often based on a fear of those who belong to a different neighborhood, religion, culture, or nation. Hatred is sometimes passed down from one generation to the next, and personal hatred comes from hurt, anger, and resentment. Deep love that has resulted in hurt or heartbreak can turn into hatred when the people involved choose to reject the opportunity to communicate their mistakes and forgive what has happened in the past.

Hatred is ugly and always causes pain and suffering. It makes people hard, disconnected, fearful, anxious, aggressive, and capable of violence, hostility, and cruelty. People sometimes hold on to hatred because it gives them a false sense of power and belonging, allowing them to feel self-righteous and superior.

Hate is disempowering, limiting, and creates stagnation. It closes people's hearts, and blocks their souls from fully expressing and experiencing the power of love, forgiveness, intimacy, and kindness. Long-term hatred rots a person's body, making him or her bitter, hopeless, and helpless. On a physical level, hatred contributes to heart disease, respiratory problems, heartburn, hypertension, warts, and lung and liver problems.

### Process to Release Hatred:

• Place your hands on the part of your body where you feel hate most intensely. Breathe into the area for a few moments while allowing any emotion to rise to the surface with little resistance.

• Relax your hands.

• Say: "Divine Healing Intelligence, using the orange-red flame of purification, please free me from the harmful grasp of hate I have carried for [insert the person or thing's name]. I ask that the orange-red flame burn away and dissolve all anger, fear, hurt, pain, and resentment that is making my body and life heavy, limited, and stagnant. Please allow me to see light and wisdom in this situation, and help me transform hatred into compassion, fear into love, disconnection into care, and spitefulness into kindness. Give me new eyes and a new point of view so that I can transform how I see this situation. Thank you."

• Repeat the word "CLEAR" several times until you feel lighter.

• Observe the orange-red light moving through your body, mind, emotions, and energy field, and begin to clear and dissolve all negative thoughts, words, feelings, memories, and images of hatred, anger, and fear.

• In order to bring back feelings of kindness and care, do the Compassion process on page 198.

## Hopelessness

People feel hopeless when they believe they cannot contribute to or change a challenging situation. When someone feels hopeless, it is common to feel like there are no choices but to give up. They cannot see a way out of their despair, thus becoming stuck in a state of limitation and bleakness.

On the other hand, a person can look at what seems like a hopeless situation and become inspired to contribute in some way, bringing hope to all involved.

Physically, hopelessness can contribute to strokes, scoliosis, nervous breakdown, narcolepsy, muscular dystrophy, measles, insanity, hernias, feeling bloated, agoraphobia, diarrhea, prostate cancer, and sleep problems.

### Process to Release Hopelessness:

• Place your hands on the part of your body where you feel hopelessness most intensely. Breathe into the area for a few moments while allowing any emotion to rise to the surface with little resistance.

• Relax your hands.

• Say: "Divine Healing Intelligence, using the orange-red sword of light, please cut me loose from all helplessness, hopelessness, and despair. Allow me to glimpse light where all seems dark, to feel hope in hopeless situations, and to take the opportunity for transformation from desperation. I ask to become aware of the bigger picture, and to be given new insights, wisdom, and opportunities to bring about change for myself and others. Thank you."

• Repeat the word "CLEAR" several times until you feel lighter.

• Observe the orange-red sword of light moving through your body, mind, emotions, and energy field, and begin to cut through and dissolve all negative thoughts, words, feelings, memories, and images of hopelessness and helplessness.

• To bring back feelings of hope and new possibilities, do the Faith process on page 199.

### Irritation—*See* Frustration.

### Jealousy

Jealousy is an extremely destructive emotion that makes people watchful, guarded, and narrow-minded. It brings distrust and fear that someone you love is going to hurt you. On an emotional level, jealousy closes a person's heart, and creates fear and tension in every part of their body. Wanting something that someone else has is based on feelings of inferiority and lack.

By harboring ill feelings toward the people of whom one is jealous, a jealous person is often controlling, self-sabotaging, and self-limiting. Usually, jealousy keeps the individual stuck in a vicious cycle of resentment, suspicion, and distrust.

On a physical level, jealousy and envy can contribute to stomach and digestive problems, heart attack, back pain, tumors, lung issues, and many other conditions.

**Process to Release Jealousy and Envy:**

• Place your hands on the part of your body where you feel jealousy and envy most intensely. Breathe into that area for a few moments while allowing any emotion to rise to the surface with little resistance.

• Relax your hands.

• Say: "Divine Healing Intelligence, using the orange-red flame of purification, please burn and dissolve all jealousy, envy, and fear from my consciousness. Help me realize there is nothing and nobody I need to envy. Nothing anyone else has takes away from what I might gain in my life. Each of us has our own path, and I need to embrace mine and be grateful for what I have. Please help me release all suspicion, control, and distrust that I am carrying. Give me the ability to let go of all resentment, ill feeling, and belief that I am lesser than others, and that I can't have wonderful things in my life. Thank you."

• Repeat the word "CLEAR" several times until you feel lighter.

• Observe the orange-red light moving through your body, mind, emotions, and energy field, and begin to clear and dissolve all negative thoughts, words, feelings, memories, and images of envy, jealousy, and fear.

• In order to bring back feelings of encouragement and support, do the Support process on page 206.

## Judgment

We all make harmless judgments every single day, whether investing in a product, crossing the road, buying a present, or hiring an employee. Conversely, many people use judgment in an unhealthy way: they judge themselves, their bodies, their appearance, their friends, their family, and so on. Judgment can also turn into discrimination, prejudice, and intolerance of others. In that case, judgment creates conflicts which can turn into arguments, anger, and hatred, and even lead to war.

Judgmental people often become controlling because they are afraid of others judging them harshly. In reality, we are our harshest critics. Judgment is often used in comparisons: he is a better student than she; she is a better sister; he is more successful; she is more beautiful, wealthy, and clever than me; and so on. Furthermore, people are usually most judgmental of people who do the same or similar things as themselves. This is because what makes us feel uncomfortable is usually an aspect of ourselves we have not connected to and integrated. It is like a mirror effect where whatever you see in someone else that you do not like, have a reaction to, or judge is usually an aspect you do not want to see, accept, or embrace in yourself. Others reflect back to you your disowned qualities. When you accept the possibility that you and another person are similar, you stop judging them so harshly and become more open, accepting, and loving.

Judging yourself or others can prevent you from fully living and embracing your life; it makes it hard to relax and enjoy the finer things. Judgment brings frustration, agitation, fear, anxiety, and stress into your life. It can lead to laryngitis, headaches, and problems with the skeletal system, respiratory system, tongue, throat, nervous system, and ears.

**Process to Release Judgment and Discrimination:**

• Place your hands on the part of your body where you feel judgment most intensely. Breathe into the area for a few moments while allowing all emotion to rise to the surface with little resistance.

• Relax your hands.

• Say: "Divine Healing Intelligence, using the orange-red flame of purification, please help me release all judgment, discrimination, frustration, anger, and agitation. Help me dissolve all stress, anxiety, and habits of self-sabotage. Allow me to learn to honor, value, and cherish myself and other people. Free me from my own and other people's harsh judgments, opinions, and attitudes. Thank you."

• Repeat the word "CLEAR" several times until you feel lighter.

• Observe the orange-red light moving through your body, mind, emotions, and energy field, and begin to clear and dissolve all negative thoughts, words, feelings, memories, and images of judgment, discrimination, and anger.

• In order to bring back feelings of love and acceptance, do the Honor process on page 202.

## Loss—*See Grief.*

## Low Self-Esteem

People with low self-esteem often feel like they are missing out on life. Those who feel unworthy and don't value themselves are overlooked for promotions, sporting activities, friendships, and opportunities. Their attitude of victimhood causes them to attract hardships and difficulties into their lives. Feeling worthless can create depression, fatigue, self-criticism, and judgment when a person holds the belief that he or she cannot contribute anything of value.

When we carry low self-esteem and unworthiness, the body tends to break down, which can lead to acne, weight problems, diabetes, genital herpes, ovarian cancer, scleroderma, ulcers, warts, and memory loss.

### Process to Release Feelings of Low Self-Esteem and Unworthiness:

• Place your hands on the part of your body where you feel unworthiness most intensely. Breathe into the area for a few moments, allowing any emotion to rise to the surface with little resistance.

• Relax your hands.

• Say: "Divine Healing Intelligence, using the orange-red flame of purification, please dissolve all thoughts, feelings, and experiences of unworthiness and low self-esteem. Help me release all victim consciousness, limitation, fatigue, and stress from my body, mind, emotions, and energy field. Melt away any hardship, difficulties, or criticism that I have attracted, and bring back my confidence, faith, and inner power. Thank you."

• Repeat the word "CLEAR" several times until you feel lighter.

• Observe the orange-red flame moving through your body, mind, emotions, and energy field, and begin to dissolve all negative thoughts, words, feelings, memories, and images of unworthiness, low self-esteem, victimhood, fatigue, and hardship.

• In order to bring back the feeling of confidence, do the Confidence process on page 198.

## Overwhelmed—*See* Feeling Overwhelmed.

## Rejection

Feelings of rejection can stay with a person for many years—to the detriment of their relationships and well-being. Often, people take rejection personally, thinking that they are not good enough, that there is something wrong with them. So, instead of going forward and changing, they give up, close down, and feel sorry for themselves.

Fear of trusting, opening up, or getting too close to people can also occur when a person has experienced extreme rejection. Most people fear rejection, and as a result, many fail to pursue their dreams and enjoy life.

Feelings of rejection contribute to many diseases and dysfunctions, such as anorexia, arthritis, multiple sclerosis, endometriosis, paralysis, numbness, cold sores, and frigidity. Such feelings can also create breakdowns, stress, nervous anxiety, and tension.

### Process to Release Feelings of Rejection:

• Place your hands on the part of your body where you feel rejection most intensely. Breathe into the area for a few moments, allowing any emotion to rise to the surface with little resistance.

• Relax your hands.

• Say: "Divine Healing Intelligence, pour your orange-red ray of purification into every aspect of my being, freeing me from all patterns of fear, rejection, self-criticism, and self-pity. Dissolve all the ways I don't feel good enough, important enough, or capable enough to live an extraordinary life. Release all stress, strain, and fear of failure from my consciousness, and bring back my inner strength and wisdom. Thank you."

• Repeat the word "CLEAR" several times until you feel lighter.

• Observe the orange-red fire moving through your body, mind, emotions, and energy field, and begin to dissolve all negative thoughts, words, feelings, memories, and images of rejection, self-pity, stress, and strain.

• In order to bring back the feelings of acceptance, do the Recognition process on page 204.

## Resentment

Resentment is deep hurt that, suppressed and unexpressed, becomes anger. It is usually directed toward a family member or someone close, and frequently comes about when you feel that you have been treated unfairly or taken advantage of.

Commonly, when people carry resentment, they hold on to it through feelings of righteousness. They have an "I'm right, they're wrong" attitude, and they choose to hold on to this feeling, believing it gives them the power to hurt someone else. In reality, it hurts them more, and produces dis-ease and discomfort in their body.

Long-term resentment can rear a host of negative emotions, such as bitterness, hurt, fear, anger, and revenge. It creates misunderstanding and distrust. If you are unable to trust, then you can never relax because, consciously or subconsciously, you are always on guard. Physically, it can lead to tumors, syphilis, osteoporosis, lupus, back pain, and more.

### Process to Release Resentment:

• Place your hands on the part of the body where you feel resentment most intensely. Breathe into that area for a few moments, and allow any emotion to rise to the surface with little resistance.

• Relax your hands.

• Say: "Divine Healing Intelligence, using the orange-red flame of purification, please dissolve all resentment, suppressed anger, hurt, injustice, distrust, and feelings of righteousness from my cellular memories, emotions, mind, and energy field. Free me from all resentment I carry for [insert the name of a person, place, or experience, if appropriate] and release any resentment or animosity they carry toward me. I ask that all negative and heavy energy associated with resentment now dissipate and vanish from my life. Thank you."

• Repeat the word "CLEAR" several times until you feel lighter.

• Observe the orange-red flame moving through your body, mind, emotions, and energy field, and begin to dissolve all negative thoughts, words, feelings, memories, and images associated with any person, place, or experience that has bound you.

• If you feel you are ready to forgive this person, then do the Forgiveness process on page 200.

**Sadness—*See* Grief.**

**Shame**

Shame is an emotion most people don't talk about much, except to occasionally say "What a shame," or "You should be ashamed of yourself." However, deep shame can stay in the body for years. Typically experienced in childhood, shame is carried over into adulthood and can have a huge effect on confidence, well-being, and success. It is connected to feelings of embarrassment and humiliation, often by the people we are the closest to, such as our family members.

We can also carry shame within our cells, from family members who have suffered humiliation in the past or from a country we have been born into, especially if the country has been through that which we are strongly opposed to, such as war. People can also feel embarrassed about their parents, religion, job, appearance, and so on.

People also feel shame if they have cheated, lied, intimidated someone, or caused pain. They often feel a sense of regret and remorse for those actions. However, unless they forgive and let go, shame can rot the body.

In particular, shame can affect the reproductive and sexual areas of the body. It can lead to conditions, such as AIDS, genital herpes, chlamydia, impotence, ovarian and prostate cancers, arthritis, compulsive eating, gingivitis, kidney stones, multiple sclerosis, urinary tract infections, and vaginitis.

**Process to Release Shame:**

• Place your hands on the part of your body where you feel shame most intensely. Breathe into the area for a few moments, allowing any emotion to rise to the surface with little resistance.

• Relax your hands.

• Say: "Divine Healing Intelligence, using the orange-red sword of light, cut me loose from all shackles of shame, embarrassment, humiliation, disgrace, and dishonor that bind me. Please help me release and dissolve all self-consciousness, self-doubt, feelings of insecurity and intimidation. Allow me to forgive all those who have shamed me and to be forgiven by all those whom I have shamed. Help me recover my self-worth, self-belief, and self-respect so that I can truly live my life with dignity and honor. Thank you."

• Repeat the word "CLEAR" several times until you feel lighter.

• Observe the orange-red light moving through your body, mind, emotions, and energy field, and begin to cut through and dissolve all negative thoughts, words, feelings, memories, and images of shame, embarrassment, disgrace, and humiliation.

• In order to bring back feelings of respect and honor, do the Respect process on page 205.

## Stress

Stress is one of the biggest problems facing Western society. Many people are experiencing increased pressure to survive, pay bills, and achieve success in a competitive environment. People complain that there are not enough hours in the day to get everything done and put extra strain on themselves to complete tasks. This means that they neglect themselves and those close to them, which causes their health and well-being to deteriorate.

Stressed people often fail to live in the present, focusing instead on future events, such as getting somewhere on time, making some deadlines, or obtaining something they want.

Stress creates tension in people's minds, bodies, and feelings, and blocks them from moving forward in life. When people are stressed, they tire more quickly, their concentration levels decrease, they feel uninspired, and they take longer to complete tasks.

Stress is a contributing factor to many physical problems, including strokes, seizures, heart attacks, immune system disorders, jaw problems, memory loss, teeth grinding, nail biting, angina, anorexia, baldness, candida, and emphysema, among others.

**Process to Release Stress:**

• Place your hands on the part of your body where you feel stress most intensely. Breathe into the area for a few moments, allowing any emotion to rise to the surface with little resistance.

• Relax your hands.

• Say: "Divine Healing Intelligence, using the orange-red flame of purification, please help me release all the ways I hold stress in my body. Inspire me to rest, nurture myself, and relax so that I can allow my body to revive and let go of tension, pressure, and strain. Every time I feel tension and stress in my body, remind me to breathe, relax, and unwind. Help me to find humor and lightness in stressful situations, and to become healthier, stronger, and more vibrant. Thank you."

• Repeat the word "CLEAR" several times until you feel lighter.

• Observe the orange-red light moving through your body, mind, emotions, and energy field, and begin to clear and dissolve all negative thoughts, words, feelings, memories, and images of stress, heaviness, and tension.

- In order to bring back feelings of rest and relaxation, do the Relaxation process on page 205.

## Stuckness

Many problems in your body and in your life occur when you are feeling stuck, inflexible, and attached to one point of view. This often takes place when the same thoughts or scenarios play themselves over and over in your mind.

When you feel stuck, everything in your life and body becomes stiff. Your creativity gets blocked. You start to experience hardship and struggle, and take on the attitude that life is hard, which in turn creates hardness in your body, mind, and emotions.

Long-term stuckness or stiffness can lead to varicose veins, sciatica, repeated strain injury, rheumatoid arthritis, paralysis, obesity, mouth ulcers, kidney problems, and a host of other diseases.

### Process to Release Stuckness:

- Place your hands on the part of your body where you feel stuckness most intensely. Breathe into the area for a few moments and allow any emotion to rise to the surface with little resistance.

- Relax your hands.

- Say: "Divine Healing Intelligence, using the orange-red flame of purification, please dissolve all stuckness, stiffness, inflexibility, blockages, struggle, and limited points of view. Help me let go of all hardness in my mind and emotions. Work with me to release patterns of strain, struggle, effort, and resistance. Please melt away all blockages in my mind, body, and emotions that obstruct my flow of energy and circulation. Thank you."

- Repeat the word "CLEAR" several times until you feel lighter.

- Observe the orange-red flame moving through your body, mind, emotions, and energy field, and begin to dissolve all negative thoughts, words, feelings, memories, and images of stuckness, inflexibility, resistance, and limitation.

• Create more flexibility in your life using the Flexibility and Movement process on page 200.

**Worry—*See* Fear.**

## *Process to Enhance Healthy Emotions*

Focus on these positive emotions and make a conscious decision to have them replace dense feelings that may have been holding you from the life you want. To do these exercises, find a quiet, comfortable location and body position. Before starting, take the time to breathe deeply for several moments. Keep a notepad and pen nearby to write down insights that may come to you in the process.

### Clarity

• Say: "Divine Healing Intelligence, infuse me with your radiant beam of clarity. Uncover any gray areas of confusion, conflict, or worry I may be feeling and dissolve these by shining your light upon them. Help me become focused and crystal clear on my life's direction, the decisions I need to make, and the opportunities I need to embrace. Illuminate my path with your brilliant wisdom so that I feel confident to ask questions and am open to receive the most empowering answers. Help me to live each day purposefully, confidently, and joyfully. Thank you."

• Repeat the word "CLEAR" several times until you feel lighter.

• Clarity is a state where your mind is free from worry and uncertainty. It requires a level of knowing yourself so that the decisions you make empower you, and make your life experience deeper and richer. When you need clarity, focus on asking yourself empowering questions, such as, *If I were making this decision from my heart and soul, for the greatest good of all, what choice would I make?* Or you may ask, *Is this the best decision for me to make?* Each person receives a response based on their perceptions, events, and experiences of their life.

## Compassion

- Say: "Divine Healing Intelligence, please pour your pink light of compassion into every cell of my body that carries the burdens of hatred, resentment, and fear. Wash away all density from my mind, body, and affairs. Help me to soften and forgive myself and others for our mistakes, ignorance, and lack of understanding. In forgiveness, allow me to find freedom from hatred, hurt, fear, and resentment, and transform these into compassion, kindness, affection, and connection. Thank you."

- Repeat the word "CLEAR" several times until you feel lighter.

- In order to find authentic compassion, imagine walking in other people's shoes. What pain must they be experiencing to be hurtful or cruel to others? Rather than react negatively toward them, which will only perpetuate the situation, find ways to heal your own hatred and fear, and transform it into compassion. Your compassion allows others to free themselves, and change how they see themselves and the situations they have created.

## Confidence

- Say: "Divine Healing Intelligence, I call on the gold ray of wisdom to awaken my inner strength, confidence, and self-worth. Help me open my heart to love, joy, and enthusiasm for life. Fill me with your light, wisdom, and faith. Strengthen my belief in myself, and support me in making my dreams a reality. Thank you."

- Repeat the word "CLEAR" several times until you feel lighter.

- Focus on your strengths. What are you good at? What do you enjoy? What makes your heart sing? Write those things down, and begin following your dreams. Every time you have a success, celebrate it.

## Encouragement

• Say: "Divine Healing Intelligence, I call on the pure white ray of honor to raise my opinion of myself, my life force energy, and my spirit. Pour your healing light into every part of me that feels lost, broken, weak, and dispirited. Surround me with encouragement, praise, inner knowing, and harmony. Bring me into a holy relationship with myself so that I can truly know my heart and soul. Thank you."

• Repeat the word "CLEAR" several times until you feel lighter.

• Focus on praise rather than criticism. Become aware of how you are thinking. Are you criticizing or encouraging yourself and others? Focus on building up your self-esteem. Be kind to yourself when you make mistakes.

## Faith

• Say: "Divine Healing Intelligence, fill me with your deep magenta ray of faith. Allow the spirit of wisdom, courage, and Divine Love to surround and uplift me. Help me to believe in myself and to develop my ability to courageously deal with challenging situations, while still having faith that I am loved and protected. Awaken the clearest and purest intentions in me so that I can use my gifts and abilities for the greatest good of all. Help me to have faith and pray for Divine Intervention, even in the darkest circumstances. Show me on a daily basis how a little faith and kindness can move mountains and transform lives. Thank you."

• Repeat the word "CLEAR" several times until you feel lighter.

• When we have faith, we tune into the unseen, mystical world we live in. We believe without needing to touch or physically see the results. There is an inner knowing that assures us that help is on its way. When we have faith, we also have the courage to follow our dreams and to make them come true. Think about what you would love to experience but have been too afraid to take a step toward.

## Flexibility and Movement

• Say: "Divine Healing Intelligence, I call on the green-white ray of rejuvenation to clear and recharge all levels of my consciousness. Please regenerate my flexibility, movement, and circulation to its full vitality. Awaken my creativity, understanding, and compassion. Allow love, healing, and abundance to flow freely into my life. Thank you."

• Repeat the word "CLEAR" several times until you feel lighter.

• In order to bring more flexibility and movement into your life, you must be willing to move your body and become flexible. A great way to do that is to focus on relaxing your body and mind while allowing inspiration to flow. Dance can help you loosen up, have fun, and free your soul. Put on some relaxing music, stand up, and imagine that you are a wave in the middle of an ocean. Allow yourself to get into the flow, and move as you focus on ease, flexibility, openness, receptivity, appreciation, acceptance, and allowance.

## Forgiveness

• Imagine the person you are now ready to forgive. Remember, you are doing the process more for yourself than for someone else, as when you forgive, you are forgiving or letting go of a destructive emotion. This does not mean that you condone any harmful words or actions from this person; you are just letting go of the pain or discomfort you are carrying that was caused by this person.

• Say: "Divine Healing Intelligence, I call on the blue-white flame of forgiveness to help me let go of all harmful ties between me and [insert the name of the person or experience that has kept you stuck]. Please release all the resentment, anger, hurt, and distrust between us. Dear [insert name] I forgive you for [state the source of your hurt or anger]."

• If appropriate, say, "I ask you to forgive me for [state what you would like to be forgiven for]. I ask that all harmful energies be dissolved by the blue-white flame of forgiveness, purifying our hearts and minds, freeing us wholly. Please fill us with Divine Love and compassion. Thank you."

• Repeat the word "CLEAR" several times until you feel lighter.

• Focus on your heart and soul. Imagine that all resentment is releasing from them. Allow the blue-white flame to dissolve all harmful ties between you, and to purify your heart and soul. When the density has released, focus on filling your heart with Divine Love and compassion. You may need to do this process several times in order to experience complete forgiveness.

## Freedom

• Say: "Divine Healing Intelligence, please re-energize my consciousness with your violet ray of freedom. Allow me to experience the freedom of choice, confidence, and self-expression. Help me become independent, make empowering decisions, and pursue my dreams. Help me live my life free of internal chains and conflict that limit my self-expression and exploration of life. Place me in an environment that gives me the freedom to discover my passion and the means to pursue it. Guide me to my own Divinity and discover my greatness. Thank you."

• Repeat the word "CLEAR" several times until you feel lighter.

• The first step to freedom is recognizing that you have a choice. Each person has the freedom to view the world from whatever perspective he or she chooses. Focus on appreciating where you have freedom, and work toward letting go of inner limitations and conflict where you do not.

## Happiness

• Say: "Divine Healing Intelligence, please shine your yellow ray of happiness into every aspect of my being, energizing, brightening, and revitalizing me. Awaken laughter, joy, and fun in my life. Bring back my optimism, inner strength, and pleasure. Sweep through every cell in my body, awakening, enlivening, and renewing it. Thank you."

- Repeat the word "CLEAR" several times until you feel lighter.

- Happiness is a choice. Make a decision to welcome happiness, joy, and laughter into your life. Ask yourself, "What am I happy about now?" Focus on joy, laughter, and fun. Many people caught up in life's problems stop nurturing themselves and having fun. Joy, happiness, and fun keep us healthy, energized, and enthusiastic. So, start planning fun things to do. Notice in every moment what gives you pleasure, even if you are stuck in traffic or standing in line at the store.

## Honor

- Say: "Divine Healing Intelligence, please flood my consciousness, emotions, and body with the pink ray of unconditional love and honor. Allow me to see, feel, and experience my true value. Awaken my sense of compassion for others, and guide me in supporting them in the best, most loving way possible. Inspire me to see my own and other people's magnificence, acceptance, and honor. Revive my inner strength, and heighten my faith in myself and my ability to make the most empowering decisions possible. Thank you."

- Repeat the word "CLEAR" several times until you feel lighter.

- Become aware of how judgments have affected your life and the people around you. Begin valuing, honoring, and supporting yourself and others to make your life and theirs a more empowering, wonderful experience. Each day, think about the way you view others. Do you appreciate and value them, and the role they play in your life?

## Innocence

- Say: "Divine Healing Intelligence, I call on the green-white flame of purity to regenerate my body, clear my mind, and uplift my soul. Please unlock all areas of my life that contain joy, laughter, innocence, and light. Free me from all negativity, shackles, and limitations. Reawaken my enthusiasm for life, and raise my consciousness from dullness to clarity and inspiration. Thank you."

• Repeat the word "CLEAR" several times until you feel lighter.

• Allow yourself to connect to and focus on that which is pure, like babies, flowers, animals, spiritual teachings. Also wear green and white for a few days, or visualize those colors bathing your body.

## Joy

• Say: "Divine Healing Intelligence, using the joyous ray of sunlight, please bring happiness, confidence, vitality, and vivacity into my life. Help me become more exuberant, energetic, and dynamic. Flood me with your light, and allow my life to flow with ease, harmony, and grace. Help me connect deeply with the Divinity of life, and have access to limitless spiritual nourishment, inspiration, joy, and love. Help me open my heart fully to experience deep warmth, affection, compassion, and openness while knowing from the depth of my soul that I am loved, cherished, and cared for. Grant me the faith to know that I am not alone and will always be looked after. Thank you."

• Repeat the word "CLEAR" several times until you feel lighter.

• People experience joy when their hearts are open to give and receive love. No matter who you are, you have the ability to contribute to others—to touch and warm their hearts. If you would like to experience more joy, focus on what you can do or say to inspire someone else, and then become aware of your heart opening. When people are joyful, they are connected to the Divine Source of love. Each day, communicate with that spiritual part of you. Listen to this Divine aspect of yourself, and allow it to guide you.

## Love

• Say: "Divine Healing Intelligence, I call on the pink ray of Divine Love and wisdom. Please heal every part of my consciousness and cellular memories where I hold fear instead of love, worry instead of peace, and anxiety instead of faith. Surround me with your loving, protective, peaceful ray of light, so that

203

I can feel safe, empowered, supported, nurtured, and loved in every situation that I encounter. Thank you."

• Repeat the word "CLEAR" several times until you feel lighter.

• Look for a blessing in every challenging situation, and remember that whatever you think about, you will attract. Focus on what you would love to happen instead of worrying about what you don't want to happen.

• Begin every day with an intention of how you would like your day to go. Say to yourself, *Today is going to be a wonderful, prosperous day.* Think of all the wonderful things you would like to create that day, and be grateful for all the opportunities that flow your way.

## Peace

• Say: "Divine Healing Intelligence, I call on the blue ray of peace and tranquility. Please bathe me in your healing light of serenity, calm, and stillness. Soothe all irritation and anger in my consciousness, and transform it into enthusiasm, balance, and passion for life. Allow me to find freedom in the stillness of my mind. Help me appreciate my life, and grow to be more dynamic, vibrant, and energetic. Thank you."

• Repeat the word "CLEAR" several times until you feel lighter.

• How would it feel to let go of all anger and negativity to discover peace and freedom? Be willing to let go of anger, and focus on peace instead. Find time for stillness and quiet where you can allow inspiration to flow to you.

## Recognition

• Say: "Divine Healing Intelligence, I call on the pink ray of love to open my heart so that I experience the joy of receiving love, appreciation, and healing. Help me recognize who I truly am: a magnificent, Divine soul. Help me treasure, believe, and trust in the Divine and hidden aspects of the universe. Allow my current relationships to heal and flourish. Bring wonderful new people into my life who will support, cherish, and treasure our connection. Thank you."

• Repeat the word "CLEAR" several times until you feel lighter.

• Focus on receiving. This means that if someone gives you a compliment, a gift, a raise, or praise, take a moment to really receive this and acknowledge yourself. Every day, begin to recognize that which is good, positive, and beautiful in your life. Do that by writing it in a journal and affirming it to yourself every morning before you get out of bed. Learn to recognize great things as they occur in your life.

## Relaxation

• Say: "Divine Healing Intelligence, please embrace me with your gentle, soothing emerald light. Allow it to flow through every muscle, bone, and tissue in my body, softening, relaxing, and calming it. Help me find peace in the chaos that surrounds me. Inspire me to take time out for myself, to commune with nature, and to revive by becoming aware of what is truly important. Allow me to find pleasure in simple things and to remember to appreciate what is valuable in my life. Thank you."

• Repeat the word "CLEAR" several times until you feel lighter.

• Become aware of how your body feels. Focus on breathing slowly and deeply, allowing every part of you that is holding stress to soften, relax, and let go. Give yourself permission to take time out, to relax, and to rest.

## Respect

• Say: "Divine Healing Intelligence, please fill my body, consciousness, and emotions with the orange ray of vital energy. Please infuse me with courage, optimism, and respect. Replenish my energy, self-worth, and self-belief. Clear the shame, pain, and density from my past and future relationships, and infuse them with light, love, honor, respect, and value. Teach me to love, validate, and cherish myself. Thank you."

• Repeat the word "CLEAR" several times until you feel lighter.

• Look at your life and become aware of where you honor, validate, and make empowering choices, and where you do not honor and respect yourself. When you are aware of the areas you need to work on, you can begin healing, changing, and transforming. Use this Respect process often to help you release shame and welcome respect.

## Satisfaction

• Say: "Divine Healing Intelligence, embrace me with your radiant gold beam of satisfaction, happiness, contentment, and delight. Allow me to feel confident that I am moving in the perfect direction for my life. Help me to recognize and celebrate all the wonderful things I have achieved, all the magnificent people with whom I have connected, and all the rich experiences I have lived. As I recognize the grandness of my life, I feel truly blessed. Thank you."

• Repeat the word "CLEAR" several times until you feel lighter.

• Satisfaction comes from celebrating life and its enriching experiences. Rather than focusing on what you don't have enough of, focus on all the things you are blessed with—even the ability to move your hands to pick up a pen, write a journal entry, read a book, or share your special gift with the world. You may simply celebrate the fact that you are alive, that the sun comes up each day, that the birds sing. Embrace and show your satisfaction, and you will see how things start to grow and develop in your life at an accelerated rate.

## Support

• Say: "Divine Healing Intelligence, please encircle me with your ray of gentle, supportive, and uplifting gold light. Infuse me with compassion, understanding, kindness, and wisdom. Help me become considerate, thoughtful, and forgiving. Transform any jealousy I feel into encouragement and happiness for other people's good fortune. As I become thankful for my own and other people's fortuity, reward me with magnificent, abundant surprises. Thank you."

• Repeat the word "CLEAR" several times until you feel lighter.

• Focus your attention on how you can support and encourage others to be their best. Concentrate on being happy for other people's success. The happier you can be about someone doing well, the more likely you will open the gateway for your own good fortune. Every day, when you are walking down the street, practice seeing everyone who passes as a great success. You may even say an affirmation, "You are a success."

## Success

• Say: "Divine Healing Intelligence, bathe me with your gold rays of success, achievement, and fulfillment. Allow me to recognize and celebrate all the success I have achieved in my life, and to honor all the people who have contributed it. Help me expand my horizons, sharpen my abilities, and prepare for the enormous opportunities that are coming my way. I ask to be a magnet for abundance, success, and prosperity and to share my good fortune with others, for the greatest good of all. Thank you."

• Repeat the word "CLEAR" several times until you feel lighter.

• Everyone has a different idea of what defines success. For some, it is about accumulating great wealth, becoming good at what they do, having children, being healthy, or having great relationships. Whatever success means for you, appreciate the success you already have in your life. It is much easier to build on success when you already have some. And even if the success is small, acknowledge it and move forward with confidence.

# IV

# The Secret Language
# of Color

For thousands of years, people have used colors for healing, entertainment, to create beauty, and to feel more radiant and alive. And colors are everywhere: in nature, our homes, our closets, and our food. This section will show you how to integrate the power of color into your own life.

As you discover the various components of each color, you can begin to use them consciously. Each of the colors contains properties of temperature, weight, and vibration. This means some colors create heat while other colors have a cooling effect. In scientific experiments where a thermometer was placed into various colored glasses, the results demonstrated that red rays give off the most heat while blue rays are the coolest.

Every disease in the body gives off a vibration, which has a color. When a complimentary color is introduced into a diseased area, it interferes with the vibration of the disease and can contribute to relief. To be effective, color healing must treat the overall cause and not merely a symptom. Combining color healing with emotional clearing processes can be extremely effective.

Colors may be used to help people heal in many ways: through visualization, clothes and shoes, food and drink, home decoration, bedding, nature, crystals, essential oils, bath salts, lamps, candles, jewelry, and makeup, as well as working with plants or flowers, painting, drawing, coloring hair, and drinking water from a colored glass that has been sitting in the sun.

In part I, you may have read about a color associated with a particular part of the body. Or you may read through the following pages and, after learning about each color, tune into your body in order to become aware of which part of your body needs what color. However you become aware of the body parts requiring attention, mentally surround each part with its corresponding color.

Another way to feel color is to rub your hands together, place them slightly apart, and visualize a color between your hands until you feel its vibration. If it is purple, you will feel heat; if it is turquoise you are likely to feel coolness. Once you feel the vibration, place your hands next to the part of your body that needs this color and take in a deep breath. Then visualize the color moving through that part of your body and healing it.

Colors can also help you open your heart, increase your energy, boost your confidence, provide clarity, relieve stress, and bring peace. I have worked with many people who have benefited from learning how to heal with colors and who now use them in every area of their lives.

Andrea, who always wore black, never seemed to have enough energy to look after her two small children. She came into my office exhausted, as if she were carrying a heavy burden on her shoulders. When I inquired why she always wore black, she said that it was the only color she had in her closet. It was interesting to observe that everything in Andrea's life also seemed black and white. I recommended that Andrea consider bringing more color into her life—in the clothes she wore, her home, the food she ate, and so forth. Amazingly, as Andrea began to wear more colorful clothes, her attitude toward life also began to change. She became more flexible, creative, and happy. I also asked her to explore using color in her visualization, and within a short time, her energy levels had increased dramatically.

Many of my workshop participants who are massage or beauty therapists visualize different healing colors while working with clients. They report that their clients often say how much more relaxed and better they feel after a session.

The steps to feel more benefits of color are simple: To experience more peace and relaxation, wear blue and white, or introduce more green plants into your environment.

To open your heart to love, you may wear orange and carry a pink crystal. To boost your energy, eat red food and wear red, orange, or gold. In order to increase your confidence, wear turquoise jewelry and blue clothes. For improved sleep, buy indigo-colored bed linen. You can even use red and gold to attract wealth, prosperity, and abundance into your life.

Consider the way you decorate your home and office, and the colors you wear. Color is just one factor, but it can be a very important one. Use the information in this section to discover the secret language of color and how it can change your life.

## The Colors

### Black

Black is a color of protection, strength, and retreat. It is connected to discipline, persistence, and respect. A gateway to new experiences, it is a test of strength and resolve. Many people experience the dark night of the soul in order to gain wisdom and emerge on the other side. Teenagers may use black as a way to rebel, and gain control and independence.

Black can help you dissolve and let go of the old so that you can welcome the new. However, too much black can weaken your body, drain you of energy, and create gloom and pessimism. It can also stop you from moving forward, keeping you stuck in limitation.

Black spots in your aura or energy field may mean that you are ill, lack energy, feel alone, or feel like a victim. It creates negativity and unhappiness.

Combine black with other colors to help you achieve your goals confidently.

### Blue

Blue creates a sense of tranquility, serenity, and peace by soothing the mind. This color calms nerves, destroys infections, and purifies your aura. It can lead people to their truth and connection with the Divine.

Mentally immersing yourself in blue rays helps protect you from dense energies and brings you back to your center. It is a color of patience, faith, acceptance, forgiveness, and independence. Blue is good for cooling, calming, reconstructing, and protecting.

Physically, blue assists with detoxifying and clearing skin problems, and brings blood back to normal when it is inflamed or overactive. Blue also has a calming effect when people feel nervous, manic, or overexcited; it can help an introverted person come out of hiding. Containing antiseptic qualities, blue helps heal burns, stop bleeding, and relieve fevers. Blue also helps to soothe nervous irritations, increase metabolism, and build vitality.

Wear blue hues to improve your memory, let go of emotional pain, and connect to your wisdom. Blue can also help improve your communication abilities, dissolve fear, and give you the confidence to speak up. Use blue to treat problems such as itching, cataracts, glaucoma, irritable bowels, burns, diarrhea, epilepsy, hysteria, laryngitis, painful periods, heart palpitations, high blood pressure, headaches, rheumatism, shock, tooth and throat issues, ulcers, varicose veins, and sunstroke.

Too much blue can leave you cold, tired, depressed, and sorrowful, however. If you suffer from poor circulation, chest infections, asthma, colds, hyperventilation, paralysis, or want to lose weight, reduce your exposure to blue.

## Brown

Brown is a color of earthiness, hibernation, nurturing, and stability. It helps us get in touch with nature, animal wisdom, and universal intelligence. Brown also helps create healthy boundaries and attain a balanced perspective. Use it to help you connect to the healing properties of nature to revive your energy and creativity.

Brown protects, supports, and provides structure. It gives access to common sense, and provides fertility, reliability, nourishment, and resilience. Brown can assist with practicality, patience, mental stability, and security, and it promotes reflection and patience. On a physical level, brown cleanses the bowels and brings about a sense of renewal.

The best way to work with brown is in a garden, or by going to the park and connecting to trees and nature. Too much brown can create dullness, fear of change and transformation, and a reluctance to express feelings.

## *Gold*

Gold attracts abundance, expands the nervous system, and increases awareness. It helps us get in touch with wisdom, profound knowledge, self-confidence, inner strength, courage, and joy.

It is a strong color to help heal all illness, and to cut us loose from feelings of frustration, inadequacy, and futility. It can also help release trauma and create a sense of well-being.

Gold can aid in treating depression, scars, digestive problems, irritable bowel syndrome, parasites, menopausal problems, and rheumatism.

A powerful protective energy, gold strengthens all fields of the body and spirit, and helps you accept what is happening in your life. Use gold for clarity, decision making, and connecting to the spiritual realm.

Do use caution, however, as gold can overpower or overwhelm the body; it should not be used to excess.

## *Green*

Green helps overcome fear, calm the body, and release frustration and anger. If you are dealing with issues from your past, use green to help bring harmony into any situation. It can also help you make wise decisions and choices.

Green helps dissolve aggression in relationships or mend a broken heart. It helps release negative patterns and beliefs, and can help you center yourself and release shock in stressful situations. If you need to relax, meditate, and heal, green replenishes energy.

Green provides hope, increases self-esteem, and attracts money and abundance. It is a color of fertility, truth, youthfulness, innocence, and healing, and can also act as an aphrodisiac to stimulate sexual energy.

Purify the blood and restore health with green; it contains antibacterial qualities. Green can also revitalize the nervous system, heart, thymus, lungs, and liver, and it can stimulate growth to heal broken bones, build muscles, and repair tissues. In addition, green aids in healing claustrophobia, agoraphobia, biliousness, headaches, high blood pressure, nervous tics, stammering, angina, back problems, asthma, colic, exhaustion, insomnia, hay fever, heart problems, laryngitis, ulcers, and venereal diseases.

On the other side, green has been linked to envy, jealousy, and superstition.

## Gray

Gray is a useful color if you are learning how to scan your body. It can help you identify blockages in your body or aura.

Gray can also provide you with information about another person's mental, emotional, and physical state, giving you an alternative point of view to deal with challenging situations that you feel are hopeless.

Too much gray can make you feel listless, drained, and emotionally empty.

## Indigo

Indigo helps with any illnesses affecting the head, eyes, ears, and nose. It stimulates your intuition, connects you with inspiration, activates your wisdom, and increases your concentration and manifestation abilities. Indigo encourages spiritual expansion and awakens the third eye, helps you to lighten up and release whatever load of responsibility you're carrying, and helps you increase memory and communication.

Indigo can awaken buried fears, find the root of a problem, and help you dissolve old stuckness. It can be useful in treating behavioral problems in children, and mental and emotional confusion in adults. It can help you release stress, give you a sense of clarity and direction in life, and encourage you to pursue the path of healing and regeneration.

Indigo can purify the blood and reduce excessive bleeding, improve your sense of smell, and act as a painkiller. It can also help treat appendicitis, asthma, bronchitis, cataracts and other eye problems, hearing difficulties, lung and throat problems, nosebleeds, sinusitis, facial paralysis, pneumonia, back pain, bone problems, sciatica, migraines, overactive thyroids, insomnia, skin complications, and inflammation.

THE SECRET LANGUAGE OF YOUR BODY

Too much indigo can make you feel ungrounded, overstimulated, overwhelmed, and unrealistic. This can lead to a lack of action resulting in feelings of disappointment and failure.

## Magenta

Magenta is the color of deepest inner knowing; it inspires truth, clarity, and faith. Magenta can also awaken your enthusiasm for life and inspire you to connect to the higher realm of spiritual guides, angels, goddesses, and saints. It can also assist you with your journey of self-discovery and spiritual fulfillment.

Magenta allows you to connect to your feelings in order to create a deeper sense of well-being. It can also help manifest your dreams. Magenta brings peace to conflicting situations and helps people come to a mutual understanding. It is a very good color to enhance organizational ability.

Too much magenta can leave you feeling stuck and reminiscing about how good things were in the past, instead of living in the present.

## Mauve

Mauve, a pale lavender-lilac color, connects you with your intuition, awakens your inspiration, and expands your spiritual awareness. Mauve can help you let go of heavy, dense energies and lighten up.

Mauve, a color of softness, gentleness, and allowance, creates a sense of peace and tranquility. It helps with eye and ear problems, improves your memory and ability to concentrate, and is useful in clearing stuckness, giving you new insights into challenging situations. Mauve is also helpful in opening the heart after heartbreak.

Too much mauve can make you feel disconnected with physical reality, light-headed, and sentimental and confused about the present.

## *Orange*

As you will have noted in part III, orange is used in most of the remedies suggested for healing unhealthy emotions because it has the ability to bring all the emotions to the surface for clearing, playing a powerful role in healing a wide range of issues. Orange also assists in treating fear, loneliness, and depression. It improves immunity and vitality, and awakens sexual and creative energy. Orange symbolizes warmth and prosperity, and creates feelings of optimism, enthusiasm, courage, determination, and spontaneity.

Orange can help people bond in relationships by teaching them how to give and receive love. It connects people to their wisdom and intuition, allowing them to experience joy and laughter. It helps people deal with loss, grief, and shock. Orange also helps release self-consciousness, shyness, and embarrassment. As a color of movement and change, it also stimulates and increases the pulse rate.

When a person has an intense attraction to orange rays, this can indicate a shock or trauma that is keeping them from moving forward or being in the present. Orange has the ability to stir up and bring old emotions to the surface for healing.

Orange assists with healing digestive, adrenal, and kidney disorders; its rays strengthen the spleen and pancreas, and aid in the assimilation of oxygen through the respiratory system. Orange can also help restore mobility to the joints, release muscle spasms, and strengthen the lungs.

Use orange to treat asthma, bronchitis, colds, inflammation, rheumatism, gallstones, gout, lung problems, mental exhaustion, tumors, and ailments of the mucous membranes and kidneys. It stimulates appetite and can help with conditions such as anorexia, intestinal disorder, bowel problems, mental breakdowns, depression, abuse, and emotional and mental paralysis. Orange helps balance hormones, aids with fertility problems, and helps the body heal.

Too much orange can create anxiety, intensify fear and worry, and keep you stuck in the past.

## *Pink*

Pink is the energy of unconditional love. It opens the heart and helps it heal through its unique ability to release emotional problems, and bring self-acceptance and tranquility. It also helps with insomnia and the manifestation of dreams.

Pink is the color of compassion, affection, warmth, friendliness, kindness, gratitude, generosity, strength, and nourishment. It releases worry, stress, and negativity and replaces them with love. Calming, restorative, soothing, and healing, pink promotes tolerance and understanding.

Use pink to work through difficult relationships with parents, children, and lovers. It helps those who suffer from low self-esteem, loneliness, and sadness. Pink also assists people during a midlife crisis by helping them let go of old patterns. It is especially good at relaxing your muscles, and releasing irritation, anger, and fear.

Pink activates your intuition, and allows you to connect with your feminine energy and spiritual beauty. It acts as a magnet that attracts people and relationships to you.

Pink can also help to heal heart problems, such as angina, heart attacks, lack of love, emotional imbalances, as well as digestive problems, anxiety, trauma, shock, stress, and a midlife crisis. It also heals arthritis; wrist problems; hand, knee, ankle and foot complications; weight issues; paranoia; abuse; depression; and exhaustion. Pink also helps with Emotional eating, heartbreak, grief, and loss. All are surmountable through the power of pink.

Too much pink can bring out sentimentality, silliness, a desire to control someone, and the tendency to be overemotional.

## *Purple*

Purple clears mental complexes and brings out leadership qualities. It creates a connection between mind, body, and soul, and brings hope and success into your life. Purple helps with your senses of vision, hearing, and smell, as well as releasing negativity and irritation.

Purple boosts the immune system and assists in the healing process. Purple helps heal skin eruptions, rheumatism, nervous tension, and problems with the bones, kidneys, lungs, and stomach. It can help lower blood pressure, calm heart palpitations, and heal concussion, inflammation, and infertility.

However, exposure to too much purple may cause a person to lose touch with reality and become depressed. It can make you feel like you are going round and round in circles without any change. The remedy for overexposure to purple is gold.

## Red

Red contains unlimited energy, heat, vitality, and power. It's a color of enthusiasm, passion, sensuality, courage, optimism, motivation, and achievement. Red draws money, new opportunities, and prosperity into your life. It also awakens your creativity and helps you achieve your goals.

Use red as a powerful healing agent for treating blood disorders and improving circulation. It has been used to heal diseases, dry up sores or wounds, warm cold areas, and reduce pain. It helps release adrenaline, and stimulates mental and physical energy. Thus, red can assist with releasing depression, hopelessness, stuckness, and immobility. Engage it as a detoxifier to dissolve toxic energies, thoughts, and feelings from your body.

Red helps you lose weight, increases your sex drive, rejuvenates your body, and restores physical vitality. It is grounding, and offers a stronger sense of self and belonging, as well as success. If you are not in a relationship, red can help you attract a partner. It also encourages shy people to come out of their shell and feel more confident.

Representing fire, growth, excitement, danger, and destruction, red gives a sense of power. It stimulates the sensory nervous system, and is beneficial to those who suffer from deficiencies of smell, taste, sight, hearing, and touch. It excites the nerves and blood to build hemoglobin. The heat that is generated from the color red is also great for relaxing contracted muscles and clearing congestion and mucus from the body.

Red can help with treating anemia, bronchitis, colds (without fever), constipation, listlessness, pneumonia, reproductive problems, tuberculosis, and paralysis.

It is advisable not to work with red if you suffer from high blood pressure, a heart condition, fever, stress, emotional disturbance, or anxiety, as it can make you feel agitated or angry.

Too much red can also cause a person to become anxious, over-impulsive, and easily irritated, frustrated, and violent. For best results, it is advisable to use red rays in conjunction with orange and blue rays.

## Silver

Silver is the color of peace and persistence. It calms nervous tension, brings serenity, and expands awareness. Silver can also strengthen the healing process and assist with purification by releasing diseases and density from the body, and flushing toxicity from the blood and tissues. Silver helps heal the kidneys and balance hormonal function, and is known for bringing clarity, protection, and grounding.

Too much silver can make you feel stuck, listless, and emotionally unavailable.

## Turquoise

Turquoise connects you to your feelings and intuition. It builds confidence, improves communication, and awakens empathy through its the ability to awaken your heart and help you discover your life's purpose.

It makes ancient wisdom available and can provide a sense of connection to your inner mastery. It is beneficial for resolving relationship problems and gives the clarity needed for important decision making. Turquoise can also help you release self-sabotaging thoughts and emotions, and find peace in difficult situations.

On a physical level, turquoise helps with problems associated with the throat and chest area. It calms nerves, releases stress, and heals emotional shock. Turquoise can also relieve fever, neuralgia, and skin problems, such as irritation and scarring. It is a skin-building color that accelerates the healing and formation of new skin.

Overuse of turquoise can create coldness, indifference, and a lack of compassion.

## Violet

Violet regenerates the nervous system, and it aids in healing insomnia, mental disorders, physical illness, and brain injury; it activates intuition, opens creativity, and increases psychic awareness. It can also help release karma and regain freedom from issues that have affected you in the past. Using violet in healing helps you value yourself and the people around you. Those open to spiritual awareness are often attracted to violet.

On the physical level, violet assists with treating epilepsy, eye injuries, kidney problems, neuralgia, rheumatism, sciatica, and tumors. Violet also aids bone growth, stimulates the spleen, purifies the blood, and calms anger and rage. It's influence balances energy and reprograms cells.

Too much violet is associated with irresponsibility, arrogance, unreliability, and other erratic behavior.

## White

White includes the entire color spectrum and heals the whole body. It is great for clearing toxicity from the body and purifying it. When treating with white, it is important to combine it with another color beneficial to the part of the body needing to be healed.

White assists with clarity and understanding. It is the color of choice, honesty, purity, protection, and reflection. It supports people reaching for their dreams, gives them courage to face challenges, and shows them the bigger picture.

Use white to create balance, replenish your spiritual strength and vision, and open up to infinite possibilities. White also has an ability to dissipate negative thoughts and feelings between people. It brings peace and comfort at the highest level.

White represents integrity, light, holiness, truth, and surrender. It softens, moisturizes, and revitalizes the skin and can be very helpful in healing skin problems. White is also cooling and refreshing, which is why people love to wear it in hot weather. White can both hide and reveal.

Overuse of white can lead to feeling depleted and washed out.

## *Yellow*

Bright, sunny, joyful, fun, abundant, fertile, and refreshing, yellow is the color of the intellect and is used for mental stimulation. It can fuel the brain, and help you think quickly and clearly. Yellow is excellent for decision making, and it boosts memory, self-expression, and creativity. It can provide clear focus with writing, reading, interviews, studying, quizzes, and exams, and it inspires new ideas that help you retain important information.

Yellow can help you let go of negative patterns from the past, dissolve pessimism, and improve self-esteem; it can help you look at and resolve deep-seated issues.

Let yellow bring happiness, self-renewal, optimism, entertainment, laughter, and inner strength into your life. Benefit from its ability to reduce stress and release nervous tension.

Yellow also helps stimulate and repair damaged cells, and is excellent for nerve regeneration. Yellow purifies the blood, removes waste products, and stimulates the lymphatic system. It soothes inflammation, clears congestion and mucous membranes, and assists with weight loss and cellulite removal.

In addition, yellow treats diabetes, arthritis, anorexia, eczema, paralysis, indigestion, toxicity release, constipation, menopausal flushes, menstrual pain, and problems with the ears, skin, kidneys, liver, pancreas, gallbladder, hormones, and spleen. Yellow is equally great for cleansing the intestines and the liver, and is helpful in the elimination of worms and parasites. A great way to take in yellow is through sunlight, flowers, and food.

Use yellow with caution, however; too much can lead to overstimulation, exhaustion, and depression.

# V

# THE SECRET LANGUAGE OF YOUR BODY SYSTEMS

Our body systems teach us lessons of empowerment, confidence, love, compassion, forgiveness, and much more. In this section, you will learn about the different systems of your body and the roles they play. You will also discover the thoughts and feelings that contribute to the breakdown of each system.

You can work with any system as a whole to restore healing by using colors, doing emotional clearing, and changing your thinking. Or you can focus on particular parts of each system and work with the processes in part I.

The more we understand our body and its specific components, the more tools we have to bring our bodies back to complete health and balance. Healing takes us through many different stages and layers of discovering who we are. Sometimes change can happen quickly, and at other times, we can experience stuckness, frustration, and chaos. Healing occurs on many levels—physically, mentally, emotionally, and energetically. Be patient and take the time to discover and empower all the different aspects of yourself.

# The Systems of Your Body

## *The Circulatory System*

The function of the circulatory system is to carry nutrition and oxygen to every system of the body through a complex network of blood vessels. It provides sustenance and nurturing to your body, and consists primarily of the heart, blood vessels, and lymphatic system.

The circulatory system begins to break down when you hold on to anger, fear, self-loathing, criticism, disappointment, heartbreak, or a loss of confidence.

Here, it's important to practice how to give and receive love.

## *The Digestive System*

The function of the digestive system is to break down food so that energy is available for the whole body to work optimally. It also absorbs waste products from the body and then excretes these as indigestible food fiber. When the elimination of food is impaired, your health can be adversely affected.

The digestive system is largely made up of the mouth, esophagus, stomach, small intestine, large intestine, rectum, and anus.

The digestive system begins to break down when you experience unresolved anger, self-sabotage, fear, indecisiveness, guilt, blame, jealousy, victimhood.

Here, you need to practice self-empowerment, creativity, self-appreciation, nourishment for your heart and soul, and how to let go of the old and bring in the new. Learn to love and honor yourself by practicing patience and tolerance.

## *The Endocrine System*

The function of the endocrine system is to produce and release hormones into the blood stream. The hormones then act as messengers that influence almost every part of the body.

The endocrine system plays a significant role in regulating emotions, behavior, tissue function, and metabolism. It promotes growth, stimulates sexual drive, and controls temperature. It also repairs damaged tissue and generates energy.

It consists of the hypothalamus, pituitary, pineal, thyroid and parathyroid glands, thymus and adrenal glands, ovaries, testes, and pancreas.

The endocrine system begins to break down when you are feeling unbalanced, stressed, emotional, stuck, confused, and frustrated.

Here, you need to practice listening to the messages your body sends you, which gives you the opportunity to create a more balanced, healthy, and happy lifestyle.

## The Immune System

The function of the immune system is to identify and eliminate viruses, bacteria, and other foreign bodies.

The immune system is made up of lymph nodes, blood proteins known as immuno-globulins, specialized white blood cells known as lymphocytes, the organs that produce these cells, and the blood vessels that transport them.

The immune system begins to break down when you feel insecure, experience inner conflict, feel pressured, push instead of allow, or feel threatened and manipulated.

Here, you need to learn how to focus within and allow the innate wisdom of your body to notify you as to when it needs to work and when it needs to rest. Focus on staying true to yourself, and have the courage to stand up for yourself and for what you believe. Practice saying no to others, as always saying yes can compromise your well-being. Aim to live in balance, and fulfill your own needs and desires before worrying about others'.

## The Integumentary System

The function of the integumentary system is to protect, nourish, insulate, and cushion the body from the harmful substances of the outside world.

The integumentary system consists of the skin, hair, nails, and certain exocrine glands.

The integumentary system begins to break down when you feel unprotected, violated, humiliated, angry, self-critical, stressed, guilty, isolated, unsupported, and guarded.

Here, you need to develop self-belief, intuition, inner resilience, openness to others, appreciation for beauty, and self-care.

## The Lymphatic System

The function of the lymphatic system is to remove excess tissue fluids. It also produces immune and antibody cells that destroy bacteria.

It consists of lymph nodes, lymph ducts, and lymph vessels, as well as the spleen, appendix, tonsils, and thymus gland.

The lymphatic system begins to break down when you are feeling vulnerable, scared, unsupported, unloved, and rejected.

Here, you need to practice courage, self-esteem, and leadership. Focus on appreciating yourself, loving yourself, and creating a supportive environment where you can feel comfortable to be creative, lively, and spontaneous.

## The Muscular System

The function of the muscular system is to endow the body with the ability to move. It also gives the body strength, flexibility, and support.

The body is made up of three different kinds of muscle tissue: skeletal, smooth, and cardiac. In order to work optimally, muscles require energy, oxygen, glucose, and other nutrients. These substances are transported to the cells during circulation.

The muscular system begins to break down when you carry excessive tension, worry, sadness, and responsibility. Too much thinking, anger, work, fear, lack of confidence, and limited support will also weaken your muscles.

Here, you need to practice building your inner strength, creating a support network, learning to relax and let go of stress, facing your fears, and learning to express your feelings.

## The Nervous System

The function of the nervous system is to supply the essential communication link between our internal and external worlds. External information is received by the sensory organs of the nervous system and is then transmitted to the brain, which passes it on to the organs, tissues, and cells so that they can adjust to changes.

The nervous system consists of the brain and spinal cord (central nervous system), and the nerves (peripheral nervous system).

The nervous system begins to break down when you experience internal and external conflict, stress, fear, strain, blame, negativity, and depression.

Here, you need to learn about relaxation, inner strength, wisdom, personal responsibility, and how to develop a sense of humor.

## The Reproductive System

The function of the reproductive system is procreation, sexual intercourse, nourishment, and life.

The reproductive system is made up the testes, prostate gland, and the penis in males; and the ovaries, uterus, breasts, and vagina in females.

The reproductive system begins to break down when you feel victimized, wounded by past relationships, guilty, ashamed, humiliated, disgusted, angry, and critical.

Here, you need to learn how to love and value yourself, forgive others, develop self-confidence, let go of negative beliefs, and learn to enjoy your sensuality.

## The Respiratory System

The function of the respiratory system is to supply oxygen to the blood while expelling waste gases. By delivering oxygen, the respiratory system enables us to generate energy, move our bodies, and grow.

The respiratory system consists of the sinuses, throat, windpipe, and lungs.

The respiratory system begins to break down when you carry feelings of loneliness, unworthiness, hate, resentment, bitterness, grief, judgment, and anger.

Here, you need to learn about compassion, forgiveness, love, hope, and trust.

## The Skeletal System

The function of the skeletal system is to provide structure and support for the body. It also protects other body systems from the external environment.

The skeletal system consists predominantly of bones, cartilage, ligaments, and tendons.

The skeletal system begins to break down when you judge yourself and others harshly, or carry feelings of betrayal, resentment, inflexibility, limitation, bitterness, and blame.

Here, you have an opportunity to become flexible, self-sufficient, kind, responsible, and empowered. You need to learn how to forgive, adapt to new situations with a positive attitude, and look for a blessing in every situation that presents itself to you.

## The Urinary System

The function of the urinary system is to pass the water within our body through a filtration process so that the different systems of the body can utilize a clean supply of body fluids. Waste products that are retained in the body lead to disease and death.

The urinary system consists of the kidneys, ureters, bladder, and urethra.

The urinary system begins to break down when you are feeling pissed off, irritated, angry, bitter, and unworthy, and also when you carry guilt, fear, and a deep-seated belief that something is wrong with you.

Here, you need to take responsibility for your actions, forgive, let go of anger, work on your self-worth, and learn to love and appreciate yourself.

# Afterword

Every day, I am thankful I can do what I love while being inspired by the courage, strength, and healing of the people who surround me.

It is impossible to express in words the gifts I have received by discovering that I can not only heal myself but also help others transform their lives. I witness incredible miracles that literally occur in front of my eyes when people realize that they need not suffer anymore—that they have the tools to heal and need only to apply them.

Through my travels, I have discovered that no matter where people are in the world they all want similar things, such as health, happiness, peace of mind, love, abundance, and freedom. It is my deepest desire that you discover all that and more.

You already have the most incredible wisdom inside yourself. All you need to do is learn how to listen and follow it.

I would love to find out how *The Secret Language of Your Body* has changed your life. Please feel free to email your experiences to me (my address is on my website, www.InnaSegal.com).

May the Divine Healing Intelligence awaken inside you and lead you to discover the secrets of your body, mind, emotions, and soul.

Till we meet in person.

*love*
*Inna*

# INDEX

# Index

# Index

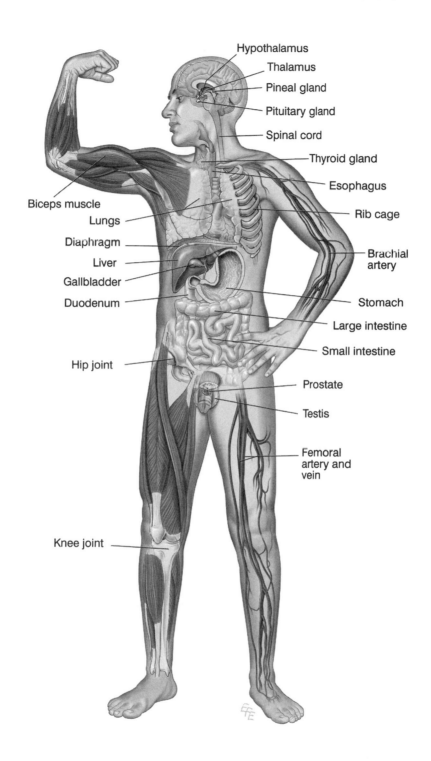

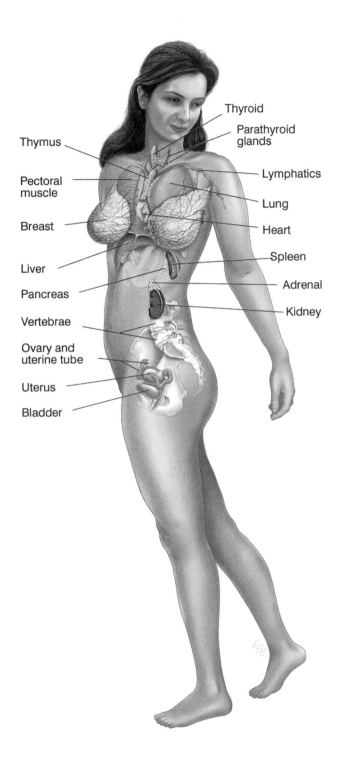

Thyroid

Parathyroid
glands

Thymus

Lymphatics

Pectoral
muscle

Lung

Breast

Heart

Spleen

Liver

Adrenal

Pancreas

Kidney

Vertebrae

Ovary and
uterine tube

Uterus

Bladder

# About the Author

Inna Segal, the creator of Visionary Intuitive Healing, is an internationally recognized healer, professional speaker, author, and television host. Inna's clients include doctors, CEOs, healthcare professionals, actors, and sports personalities.

Inna is a gifted healer and a pioneer in the field of energy medicine and human consciousness. She can *see* illness and blocks in a person's body by intuitive means, explain what is occurring, and guide people through self-healing processes.

When Inna was a teenager, she suffered from severe back pain, which continued to deteriorate despite visits to doctors, chiropractors, and other healthcare professionals. By her early twenties, Inna's pain was so intense that for weeks she was barely able to walk.

In an incredible twist of fate, Inna, while meditating, discovered an unusual way of communicating with her body. By tuning in to her back and releasing all the pain and negative emotions, she was able to heal herself.

Inna Segal dedicates herself to assisting others in their journey of self-healing and empowerment. Her practical healing techniques, healing frequency, web presence, and radio and television appearances are changing the lives of millions of people all around the world.

For further insight on Inna Segal, please visit www.InnaSegal.com.

# Resources Available from the Author

## Visionary Intuitive Healing Audio Programs

*Create Perfect Health*

*Success, Money & Prosperity*

*Affirmations for Happiness, Confidence & Wellbeing*

*Lose Weight Fast*

*Nine Chakras: The Secret to Health, Clarity & Freedom*

*Peaceful Sleep*

*Accelerated Learning & Memory Enhancement*

*Healing Your Inner Child*

*The Secret Language of Your Emotions: Volume 1*

*The Secret Language of Your Emotions: Volume 2*

*Healing Meditations for Children* (Raphael Alexander Segal)

*Right Now*—inspirational songs

*Freedom from Pain*

*Experience Youthful Clear Skin*

*The Secret Language of Color* (card deck)

*The Secret Language of Your Emotions: Volume 1 and Volume 2*

## The Secret of Life Wellness

### *The Essential Guide to Life's Big Questions*

In *The Secret of Life Wellness*, Inna Segal goes beyond physical healing to demonstrate that life wellness reflects health wellness. By answering twenty-one of life's biggest questions, Segal guides you through every stage of your personal well-being and invites us all to look within to find answers. From losing weight to raising confident children and dealing with loss, Segal covers the full spectrum of human challenges.

With simple wisdom and easy and impactful exercise that can be integrated into one's day-to-day life, Segal clears away the complexity to offer "must have tools" for healing, transformation, and evolution.

Discover life-changing secrets to enable you to:

- Develop your intuition
- Create harmony in your relationships
- Attract money and success into your life
- Deal with challenging emotions
- Attract and understand soul mates
- Dramatically improve your health
- Discover your soul's purpose
- Embrace your shadow side
- Use your energy centers to heal and evolve
- Experience unconditional love
- And much more

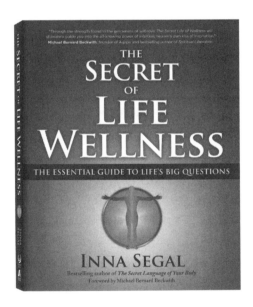

## The Secret Language of Color Cards

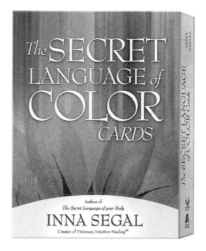

*The Secret Language of Color Cards* offers the key to unlocking the extraordinary healing power of color. Featuring an easy-to-use guidebook and 45 vibrant color cards—each infused with a unique healing vibration—it's easier than ever to bring joy, harmony, balance, and wellness to all aspects of your life.

Combining tips and information on colors with powerful healing processes and affirmations, this practical, hands-on card deck can help you restore your body to its natural state of health and harmony. Discover the success of **scarlet**, **amber's** special creative powers, **jade's** call to action, and **plum's** ability to help you overcome any challenge that comes your way. Whether seeking daily guidance, physical healing, or emotional well-being, these beautiful cards spanning the color spectrum, offer intuitive, inspired messages that will help you live each day with the power to create positive change.

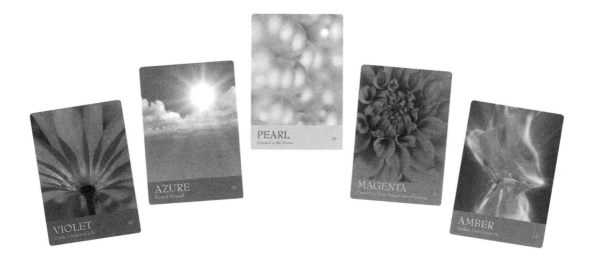

# FREE AUDIO DOWNLOAD

**Visit www.beyondword.com/innasegal/ and http://books.simonandschuster.com/Secret-Language-of-Your-Body/Inna-Segal/9781582702605 for a free audio download with Inna Segal speaking about tuning into your body.**

*Track 1—Introduction*
Inna explains how to utilize the free audio processes for the greatest results. Listen to this introduction before you participate in the two interactive processes. Each process is unique and powerful, and was developed from Inna's workshops, her work with private clients, and her own healing experience.

*Track 2—Exercise for Tuning Into Your Body*
This is a process for tuning into your body, which is similar to the one Inna used to heal herself. This process can assist you in discovering the cause of any physical or emotional challenges you may be experiencing, and guide you to activate your healing abilities to free your body from tension and pain.

# FREE AUDIO DOWNLOAD

*Track 3—Exercise for Healing Your Stuck Emotions*

This process is designed to help you let go of any stuck or unpleasant emotions you may be feeling. This track was taken from Inna's *Freedom from Pain* audio program.

---

Do not listen to these audio processes while driving a vehicle or operating machinery.

Listen to this audio program when you can close your eyes and relax completely.

All Visionary Intuitive Healing audio processes contain healing frequencies transmitted by Inna Segal.

35 Minutes. ℗ & © 2010 Inna Segal. All rights reserved.

All vocals by Inna Segal. Original Visionary Intuitive Healing music by Phillip Gelbach and Paul Morris Segal.